YOUR WEALTH IS YOUR HEALTH

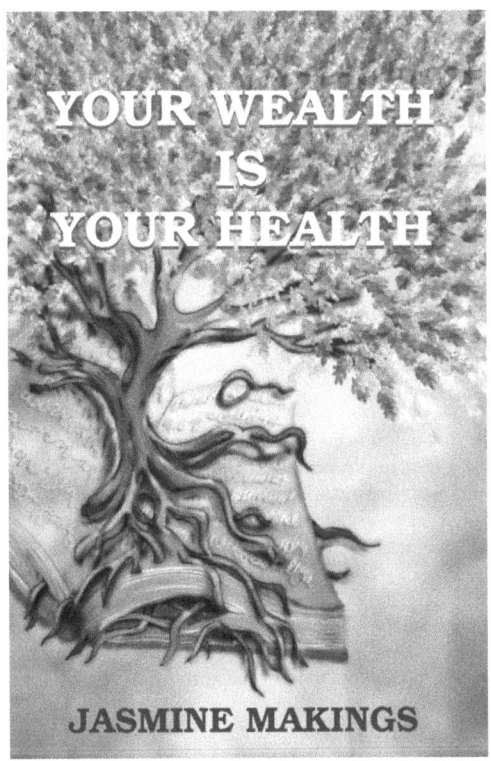

Jasmine Makings

Copyright © 2015

The moral right of Jasmine Makings to be identified as the author has been asserted by her in accordance with the Copyright, Designs and Patents Act 1988. All rights reserved. No part of this book may be used or reproduced, stored in a retrieval system, or transmitted in any form, or by any means electronic, mechanical, recording, photocopying, or in any manner whatsoever without permission in writing from the author, except for the inclusion of brief quotations in a review.

National Library of Austraalia Cataloguing-in-Publication entry (pbk)
Creator: Makings, Lesley J., author.

Title: Your wealth is your health / Lesley J Makings.

ISBN: 9780994288400 (paperback)

ISBN: 9780994288417 (ebook)

ISBN: 9780994288424 (hardback)

Subjects: Health

         Nutrition.

         Natural foods.

Dewey Number: 613.2

Book Cover Layout: Laila Savolainen (Pickawoowoo Publishing Group)

Publishing Consultants - Pickawoowoo Publishing Group

All rights reserved.

No part of the book may be transmitted or reproduced by any form or means, either mechanical or electronic, including recording and photocopying, or by any known storage and retrieval system, without the written consent of the author, except in the case of short quotations being used in a review

This book is designed to provide information and motivation to readers and is not intended as a substitute for the medical advice of physicians. The eclectic practitioner will offer treatments that are for you, the person and not treat a condition. This book does not take the place of a professional consultation. If you need professional assistance, you should seek the services of a competent holistically trained health care professional or medical professional.

Neither the author nor the publisher shall be responsible or liable for any person or entity with respect to any loss or damage caused, or alleged to have been caused, directly or indirectly, by the information contained in this book. Neither the author nor publisher shall be responsible for physical, psychological, emotional, financial or commercial damages, including, but not limited to, special, incidental, consequential or other damages. Our views and rights are the same. You are responsible for your own choices, action and results.

Some names and identifying details have been changed to protect the privacy of individuals.

www.jasminemakings.com

*I dedicate this book
For the Glory of Good Health
And with it
Good Life*

CONTENTS

ACKNOWLEDGEMENTS	v
CHAPTER 1 GOOD HEALTH NATURALLY	1
CHAPTER 2 STEP 1 - UNDERSTAND WHAT YOU ARE EATING	18
CHAPTER 3 STEP 2 - WHAT WE SHOULD AND SHOULD NOT EAT	35
CHAPTER 4 STEP 3 - CHILDREN	58
CHAPTER 5 STEP 4 - HOW CHEMICALS IN OUR TOILETRIES AND COSMETICS AFFECT OUR HEALTH	66
CHAPTER 6 STEP 5 - HOW CHEMICALS IN THE HOME AFFECT OUR HEALTH	75
CHAPTER 7 STEP 6 - FIRST AID – HELP YOURSELF WITH KITCHEN CUPBOARD AND NATURAL REMEDIES	83
CHAPTER 8 MORE CASE STUDIES	92
A FEW TREATS!	102
REFERENCES	108

ACKNOWLEDGEMENTS

- To my very special friend whose love and teachings have changed our lives and to the love which guided us to her.

- To my husband Brian for his love, trust and belief in me, and my children who have travelled this journey with me for many decades.

- To my clients who have given permission to use their testimonials.

- To Prof Dr Shirley Mcilvenny of The Food Coach Institute of Australia for her belief, encouragement and support.

- And my friends and family who have put up with many hours, if not years, of earache listening to me!

- To Julie-Ann and the team at Pickawoowoo Publishing for their professionalism and guidance.

CHAPTER 1

GOOD HEALTH NATURALLY

I want to prove to you, that living food is medicine and show you the healing power of your own body, and that your body is your best healer.

Some people find it hard to believe that eating living food can restore their health and even reverse chronic disease, but I tell you, it can work like magic!

It is a fact that our body replaces itself every seven years, some parts in weeks, some in months and some in years. Your current body's health is largely the result of what you have been feeding it and how you have been treating it in previous years. Therefore isn't it logical that the 'quality' and 'health' of our next body, eyes, liver, skin, heart, bones, etc will depend on what quality of food we are feeding it now? Even the brain, which requires a lot of good oils can benefit too. Therefore your health is very much in your hands!

I look back over the past forty years and see how people's health has deteriorated and is continuing to do so. Chronic disease, including cancer, is continuing to increase and the lives of our children and grandchildren are more and more threatened every day. For their sake and that of future generations now is the time to look at what has gone wrong, take a U-turn and protect the future health of generations to come.

My experience and knowledge and proof of making this U-turn is what I am sharing with you now. A logical and simple way of making those changes crucial to your health and wellbeing. This is not an idea, this is fact and I hope to prove that to you – as I have to many people over several decades. In this book I shall share with you case studies and letters from some of those people. You will see how quickly you and your family will benefit long term from making small changes. No 'special' diets, no fads, rather a re-education and understanding of a different way forward which, when on this path, you will not want to turn back when you realise and experience the benefits.

I would ask you, as I have done for many years, to share, to pass on what you learn from this and help as many people as you can to understand they have the power to change their life and their health.

THE ESCALATION OF CHRONIC DISEASE AND CANCER

Why are we seeing a constant increase in chronic disease and cancer, even in children, in spite of the $billions on research?

I look back over my lifetime and I can say without a doubt from the 1960s I have seen a huge decline in the quality and production of our food supply. As a child we had a local co-operative which was like a mini-supermarket with basic items of tinned foods, cereal and household products. Our food supply was largely sourced from the local butcher, baker and green grocer, and all of our meals were made fresh.

I believe the mid to late sixties was a time in England – and probably the rest of the Western world – when women started to want more education and careers. At that time there were very few professional women. Most mums were at home waiting for their children to come home from school and husbands from work, and they had time to prepare fresh food every day. This is no criticism or judgement; I have been a working mum. But let's look at the pattern of what happened back then which resulted in where we are now. The busier mums became working and running homes the greater was their need for 'quicker ways of doing things'. The food industry latched on to this and marketed more convenience foods.

FOOD ADDITIVES

Of course for food to sit on supermarket shelves for weeks, months and even years, something has to be added to stop them rotting, to make them look attractive to the eye, to make them taste okay etc. So, artificial preservatives would enhance the shelf life, artificial colours would restore some appeal after processing methods destroyed the colours, and artificial flavours would be added to restore some flavour to what is likely to be flavourless. It eventually became the norm that a lot of mums worked and the demand grew. We created that demand; the food industry just took advantage of it. It is now in our hands to change that! As people have become more health conscious – to some extent anyway – you will be aware that supermarkets now market 'healthier options' such as low sugar, low fat. We can be very much influenced by the marketing techniques but unfortunately this is what they are. It is our responsibility to check our labels and ingredients and really understand what we are eating. Don't be misled by the marketing of food products. This will be covered in chapter one.

Therefore, I have seen over the decades a total change for the worst as far as our food sources and diet are concerned. We have gone from most of our food being prepared and cooked at home to too many convenience foods, imported foods, junk foods and ultimately to a huge change in the balance of fresh foods to dead foods. At the same time, and no coincidence, began the rapid increase of chronic disease and cancer.

Alongside these changes I have seen the increase of chemicals in our lives – toiletries, household products, food and agricultural chemicals, and more and more dependence on medicines etc.

Is there any wonder immune systems are weakened under the bombardment of all what is not good and natural. Once upon a time our immune systems had to deal mainly with viruses and bacteria but now it has to deal with thousands of chemicals as well. Our immune systems even see a lot of our food now as alien, and it is so overwhelmed that in many cases it has turned upon itself (auto-immune diseases).

Research is not finding the answers we would wish because I believe it is looking in the wrong place as far as chronic disease is concerned!

We don't catch these diseases from someone else; our body manifests them because something is wrong, something is not working, and something is out of balance! So don't search for something external like a pill to cure the problem, look internally, invariably what causes also cures! i.e if wrong food and bad diet are the cause of the body not working properly, then good diet and good food can help reverse the problem.

Consider the following:

After one of my talks in 2013, an elderly gentleman approached me and asked me if I could help his wife. The husband said her specialist had told him there was nothing more they could do for her. He said to me they are just waiting for her to die! This lady was indeed very sick with multiple health problems; she could barely eat anything without being in pain and was invariably rushed to hospital. She was on the verge of kidney dialysis and was diabetic, had pancreatitis and many other health problems. A liquid diet was the only way initially to get those vital healing nutrients into her body.

Testimonial - July 2013

> *My first appointment with Jasmine Making was the start of better changes for me.*
>
> *When I was sixty I thought I was healthy but then everything seemed to happen almost all at once.*
>
> *First I had breast cancer, followed by a heart attack and a Bypass. Then Diabetes 2, removal of my gallbladder and a hernia repair. Along the way there was Chronic Kidney disease and Pancreatitis. All in the space of 16 years.*
>
> *My second home became the hospital. I lost weight, energy and hope. My favourite house clothes were night wear and slippers. The only time I went out was if I had a medical appointment. Life was a bore.*
>
> *NOW eight weeks after seeing Jasmine my life has changed so much. I am now coming back to wanting to be active again and taking an interest in myself and in other people. I no longer just want to be alone and be miserable.*
>
> *My regular blood test has already shown improvement with my Sugar levels so that my Doctor has halved that medication. My kidney function*

has stabilised so that I am no longer dreading the time when Dialysis could be the only option for me, and in general the whole of the tests have indicated an improvement.

I have always loved a variety of food and at first I wondered if I would be able to keep to the initial food plan, but soon I got a routine for myself, and with Jasmin's encouragement it is now second nature for me and I would not have my life any different.

I cannot express how generous Jasmine has been with her time and information. Every step of the way she has guided me and not overloaded either my mind or my system, everything has been done so that I have never felt pressured in any way whatsoever, and I am so thankful to her for the way that I now feel better than any time I have for many years. I can recommend her as a Food Coach to anyone and I would encourage anyone with health problem, or without current problems, to take heed, and with her guidance to Get Healthy.

2/11/13 continued

It is now 10/12/2013, eight weeks since I wrote the first recommendation for Jasmine, not long at all really.

It is now officially medically right for me to say that I am no longer a Diabetic person. No more Metaformin just good food. The Kidney consultant who I see was surprised, although eight weeks ago he did halve the medication. I did ask if there was a test to give me a result so that I know how my Pancreas is now doing and his reply was to me: (omission) "If your Diabetes is no longer a problem for you then both your Kidneys and Pancreas must also be improving." Really good news.

Now I know that what Jasmine has been working with me for is definitely right. I also feel ready now to stretch myself more and to start to feel part of the human race.

Once again Jasmine, THANK YOU most sincerely.

Margaret

(Permission given to print)

One of my most recent e-mails from this lady, who is 76 years old, was to tell me that she 'had put her name down' for tai chi and a computer course! She never fails to surprise me!

There are many good 'specific' diets where one can vastly improve their health, such as eating raw for 30 days, juicing for 28 days etc. but doing 'specific' diets can be very overwhelming for sick people, and what happens when they have done their 30 or 28 days or whatever? What then? What do they eat? The way forward has to be re-education, learning again what is good for our health and what isn't, and apply that principle every day of our lives, forming new habits and knowing what we are eating and why we are eating it. This lady has been a great inspiration to me and to many others. If someone so sick can get out of bed and make herself simple healthy food and drink anyone can!

INTRODUCTION

Many times over the years it has been suggested I should write a book, and my response has always been that there are thousands of books out there telling you everything you need to know about food, diet and health. Then one day, in early 2013, I felt I had to write down what I knew to be true.

The time is right, the world is sick and people are hungry to help themselves. I realised that these days' people are so busy they don't have the time to spend years researching, as I did, to find the answers. They need them now. For me this journey started forty years ago, and some thirty years ago I began studying and researching what nature has to offer us to be well and keep well. Every day I learn something new and it is a never ending journey. What nature has given us to take care of ourselves, to keep us well, sustain us, heal us and repair ourselves is beyond wonder. It is really so simple!

I wish to say at the outset that I have never taken any risks as far as my family and others are concerned, always getting medical checks if I was in any doubt. After obtaining a diagnosis from the doctor, I then had informed choices to help me decide whether I gave my family medication or treated their symptoms naturally. I did not see any point in adding more toxins to a body which was trying to fight off toxins from attacks on the body, especially in the case of colds, sore throats, tummy bugs and common everyday ailments.

A few years ago I did a series of six workshops, one a week, which was supposed to be for one hour but people got so absorbed in what I was teaching, sometimes we could be two to three hours. These workshops gave me the ideas on how to present a book which would 'bring everything together' in simple terms. Hence this book is a six-step guide to improved health. The crux, as I often mention throughout the book, is removing toxicity starting with avoiding chemicals in food and drink and other areas of our lives, and feeding the body with a lot more nutrients. Today's Western diet is full of processed carbohydrates and sugars, not enough protein and little room or time for lots of fresh food.

Our body is attacked from many directions with chemicals, whether in food, on the skin, by inhalation etc. The workshops' guide gave the attendees an insight into the areas of nutrition and hazards to health so they could start making adjustments to protect themselves and their families and embark on a healthier way of eating. I also gave them a kitchen cupboard guide for everyday ailments, which has been our natural pharmacy at home for thirty years. I want this book to be as practical and usable as possible. There are many books which are technical and detailed on the many subjects connected with food and health. I am not going into the 'nitty gritty' of antioxidants, minerals, vitamins and dissecting what foods are broken down into what etc. Neither is it about diets which invariably don't work. Neither is it about spending a fortune on vitamin pills and potions. This is about rolling the sleeves up and getting on with taking responsibility for our own health, eating the right foods and taking precautions to protect ourselves and our family. A change in thinking, permanent thinking, is what is needed!

Some people make gradual adjustments over time, whilst other 'sweep clean', and they are the ones who feel amazing benefits very quickly as you will see from some of the case studies mentioned throughout the book. It goes without saying that if you are continually getting symptoms, are tired, lethargic or have a chronic disease and you want to see results, then more rapid changes are needed.

Don't forget, symptoms are 'signals' from the body that something is wrong. To ignore the signs or to take medication to 'suppress' the symptoms is not going to make the problem go away, even if it makes you feel better for a while. Only getting to the cause and dealing with it gets long-term results. I take this approach whether I am working with chronic disease, or headaches. Apparent 'cures' can be achieved in many ways but unless the root cause is dealt with, something else will manifest again sooner or later.

MY STORY

We don't stop to think our experiences in our life from when we began our journey on Earth might be preparing us for things to come, maybe preparing us for the reason why we have been given this life. It is only when we look back and see the pieces of the jigsaw slotted together that it may occur to us.

I was born in the middle of the 1900s and named Lesley Julie Smith, a time when a doctor's word was gospel and unquestioned. We lived in a small mining village called Hemsworth in West Yorkshire, England, where grandparents, aunts, uncles, cousins and the rest lived in the same vicinity raising their children in a close-knit family atmosphere – which has its good points, but not perhaps for the new generations who wanted to spread their wings. Thankfully, my mother was very keen for me to experience all the things she never could, and that included an education, working and spreading my wings (well within reason)!

In those days, all family doctors seemed to be dedicated people who personally knew grandparents, parents, siblings and children – generations of each family – and were indeed highly respected, caring people who knew more of your family history that you did. It was no trouble to turn out late at night to see a patient so there was always continuity, which was very comforting and assuring. Of course, in those days they also had far fewer people to look after!

Mum was very suspicious of the new medications called vaccinations which were offered when we were very young, and she declined to participate in this unknown procedure, even though later in life she took every medication the doctors prescribed for anything and everything else. This is what they did and what I did, that was until one day when mum was crying out with back pain and could not get out of bed. Mum's back problem had been going on for a while, so on this occasion, late one evening, I called out the doctor to visit. I was told that mum had had X-rays and there was nothing wrong with her back, she just had a low pain threshold! I was not happy with this diagnosis. Pain is a signal not to be ignored.

I was twenty at the time; just married, working with the West Yorkshire

Police, but on Saturdays I still did a job which I had done from school days for pocket money i.e. hairdressing! It was there I heard about some 'quack' in a nearby town who 'fixed backs'. I asked for an address but was told if I went to see this person, on no account must I let the family doctor know or he would strike us off his register and we would not get medical help!

As soon as I could get mum out of bed, with great difficulty, I managed to get her into a car and off we went to see this person called an osteopath. What I witnessed was beyond belief to me. He examined mum's spine, told her she had protruding discs, one in her neck and one in her lower back, and with a twist of the neck and an adjustment on her lower back, she stood up straight, pain free and could bend down and touch her toes better than she had done for years (she was 46 at the time). The only reason I mention this incident is because this was my first experience of 'another way', something contrary to what I had been lead to believe! It certainly was a significant step in changing my way of thinking.

Well of course we didn't tell the doctor, but it did raise a lot of questions in my mind, which set me on my forty-year journey in the search and study of 'what nature had provided for us to keep well and to heal'. Whilst still working in my full-time job in 1977-79, I did a two-year Yoga Teacher Training Diploma with The British Wheel of Yoga. Yoga helped me in my stressful job so I wanted to learn what I could do to be able to help others. This training was my first introduction to harmful foods such as white flour, white sugar, wrong fats etc. Here my appetite and thirst for more knowledge about food started and the passion to learn more from wherever I could. I later self-studied homeopathy, herbs, kitchen cupboard remedies and anything that nature had provided for us to heal our body and prevent ill health. I soon began to implement this knowledge into my daily life. I learnt there was so much help in my kitchen cupboard which could sort out every day sniffles, sore throats, tummy bugs and headaches, and which didn't weaken the immune system!

Of course, family, friends, neighbours, work colleagues got a lot of earache from me talking about my findings, and people soon started to ask for help. Hence my sharing and working with people near and far to help restore health and teach prevention through diet and natural and kitchen cupboard remedies which had been around for perhaps hundreds of years.

I had friends in various positions in the medical profession who worked at our local General Hospital and I was told that when they get emergency cases such as children with meningitis, some children have had so many antibiotics in their young lives that it is difficult to find one which works in such an emergency. I found that quite disturbing. I think my children, now in their thirties, have had perhaps one antibiotic in their lives as I always found natural ways of helping common ailments.

I knew from a young girl that I wanted to be a teacher. Then instead of going to teacher training college I took a job with the police and then later went into industry. As previously mentioned, in my late twenties I had the opportunity to become a Yoga Teacher. Diet was part of the two years' training, but I didn't realise the importance of it at the time. Little did I know that my new Teaching Diploma was a door opener and an accreditation for the future which allowed me to teach about diet and health in later years. It seems to me if you are inspired to do something, sooner or later it will come to fruition. It is said your 'inner passion' should not be ignored as it may well be the reason you are here. The knowledge I gained over many years regarding health, healing, diet and nature's help which started as a passion for my family's health became a very intense passion to help mankind do a U-turn from the decline in health which continues to be with us today.

In the 1980s, I met the most wonderful lady who became my help, guide, friend and mentor. My friend was born in Krakow, Poland. She has the most amazing knowledge of nature, food and natural remedies, perhaps some of which will not even have been heard of today. More importantly she taught me how to read food labels and to understand what effect these additives had on our health. She has been a beautiful example to me too on 'how to live life', the right attitude, speaking and thinking from the heart, and how to be kind, compassionate, joyful and grateful. I am forever grateful to my friend whom I still lean on today. I call her my angel on earth, and my life and that of my family has changed for the better since we met.

Some of what I have been witness to first-hand is quite remarkable and I feel very privileged to be able to share my knowledge to help so many.

So for over thirty years I have been working in the field of 'natural health', against convention and belief systems, especially in England, where it is still difficult today to find 'natural or complimentary' therapists. Today, I live in Australia where there is an abundance of complimentary help but, unfortunately, many of the medical profession are still not receptive to integrating complimentary medicine/treatments, nor in accepting that bad diet is the cause of so many ills. I have however raised their eyebrows on some occasions!

A few years ago, I woke up one morning and I couldn't move the thumb on my right hand without it creaking and feeling very painful. My first thought was that I had inadvertently knocked my hand on something but when there was no improvement I decided to get it checked out, realising that over many years of typing, playing piano I could have a bit of wear and tear. The X-ray was clear and the doctor could offer no explanation. Making no progress with what the problem was I consulted another doctor who quoted some Latin name which in layman's terms meant 'trigger finger'. I was told a cause was not known and neither was it curable but that surgery would release the ligament which had become entrapped in a thickening sheath. I was given a letter to see a surgeon and I left the doctor's surgery in disbelief. It was suggested here that my only port of call was surgery. No known cause, no cure, but cut! As I knew what I was now dealing with, I set to work with my healing oils (organic castor oil also known as Palma Christie, or The Palm of Christ). Within a week, all was well, it was back to normal. Coincidentally, sometime later, I had a friend with the same problem and suggested she try my treatment and sure enough within a week all was well. It was some two years later when I saw the first doctor again and he asked how my hand was after the surgery. Well after twiddling my thumb in front of him for a few seconds to show it was fine, I revealed I had not had the surgery but healed it myself with a particular healing oil massage and compress.

I am also reminded of a few years ago, my mother, at the time in her late seventies had a bad nosebleed which would not stop. After several failed attempts to stop the bleeding she was admitted to hospital. One week later the problem had not been resolved and of course she was fed up and wanted to go home. I visited the hospital and took with me a natural remedy that I felt confident would stop the bleeding. Being courteous I ask the Doctor in charge of my mother's ward if I could try my natural remedy. I was told NO! Well when they had disappeared from view I started to treat my mum with the remedy. The remedy was homeopathic Arnica.

Some years previously I did a Homeopathy in the Home course. The Homeopathic Doctor I trained with told us a true scenario. She was with her daughter-in-law for the birth of her baby and after the birth the lady in question was haemorrhaging. It was a home birth and the midwife was concerned. The Homeopathic Doctor treated her with Arnica to stop the bleeding, and it did.

I sat with my mum in my lunchbreak from work for about one hour giving her the remedy every fifteen minutes, then asked her to continue for another hour. She never seemed to have faith in my 'natural' approach but was so fed up on this occasion she did as asked. That evening the bleeding stopped, the wound was cauterised and she was home the next day. I love homeopathy, I have used it in my home for my family for some 25 years or so. I will talk more about the remedies I use at home later in the book.

Do remember this was a nose bleed; it wasn't anything serious, just a nuisance. How beneficial it would be to all if medical science and complimentary treatments (which go back thousands of years before ever medical science came into being) could be brought together? I make this comment specifically because while watching an independent documentary recently on the Gerson therapy a medical professor commented that this complementary stuff is a newfangled idea! I had to smile!

Trying to help people 'naturally' in England was not easy, sometimes frustrating, while the tools I had were limited i.e. a small book on the dangers of food additives and my own knowledge! People were used to taking medication for every ache, cold, itch, tummy upset, allergies and so on and the quality of tools I had was supermarket food! Even most of the fresh food came from overseas and could be somewhat nutritionally diminished. However, what amazing changes I saw and experienced when I could get people away from tins, packets, bottles, processed foods full of additives and onto fresh food. Asthma, constipation, migraines, haemorrhoids, digestive disorders, nausea and so many other common ailments started to disappear. I remember one lady had to have iron injections and sometimes transfusions but when I encouraged her to take a certain food rich in natural iron, i.e molasses; she no longer needed the medication.

Moving to Australia in 2005, saw another huge change for us, not only in the quality of life we could enjoy largely due to the climate, but the amazing abundance of fresh local produce was like a dream to me, and all of this medicine to work with, I couldn't believe it. I also met and now communicate with medical doctors who embrace complementary treatments, diet and natural ways of helping people alongside medical science.

Fellow Australians, protect what we have here. Support our farmers, protect the land; we are so privileged to have them and their produce. Just remember if we were cut off from the rest of the world with some unforeseen circumstance, we have our own food and medicine and do not have to rely on other countries for it. We are self-sufficient.

My years in this wonderful country have also led me to further study in nutrition, food as medicine and remedies, and Reiki. I wanted to understand how energy affects the body's healing capacity and also how food can be directly linked to chronic disease.

A chance meeting with Professor Dr Shirley Mcilvenny of The Food Coach Institute of Australia further enhanced my knowledge and a deeper understanding of the link between specific 'foods' and ill health, particularly chronic disease, and gave me the much desired communication link with medical professionals who understand and embrace the need for good diet. I became her first Australian graduate in Food Coaching.

THE BEAUTY OF FOOD

My view of food is quite simple, you either eat living food or dead food and what you choose will reflect in your body and your health.

Living whole food is plucked or picked and eaten when ripe; preferably uncooked or lightly cooked if necessary. This is the most nutritious food. Once cut off from its life source, i.e. the minute it is picked it starts to die and diminish in nutrients. So our best quality, most nutritious food, is local food and preferably organic. Food from elsewhere can be picked months before the food is fit for consumption then instead of 'naturally' developing to ripeness it is stored, sprayed, delayed in completing its cycle until it gets to its destination, which in some case I understand can be six months or more. So often the so called 'fresh food' you think you are eating is actually old food and developed 'unnaturally'.

Dead food to me is anything in tins, bottles, packets, cartons, bags and tampered with by humans, and it is usually full of additives to stop the food from decaying and going discoloured. Harmful flavours will then be added as there is no natural taste left because of the processing. Not only does this food have little or no nutrition but is actually harmful because of the multitude of chemicals added.

Back in the 1920s Dr Max Gerson said chronic disease and cancer was caused by toxicity and nutritional deficiency. He recognised that immune systems were overworked from the bombardment of toxins, in food, in homes, gardens, the environment etc. and that they could no longer work efficiently and therefore were not able to protect us and deal with attacks on the body as they should. With nutritional saturation and at the same time helping the body to offload the many toxins, the immune system starts to function properly again. The reason I agree with him entirely, not just because of the worldwide proof of his help and reversal of many chronic diseases and cancers naturally for almost a century, but because in my thirty years plus experience, when a person starts to remove 'dead', toxic food from their diet and starts to eat living fresh foods, amazing thing starts to happen.

Look at this example from one of my many clients.

Testimonial

A middle aged gent came to see me saying he wanted to prevent health problems. He knew he was overweight and on a slippery slope health wise. He guessed he would have high cholesterol and possibly heading for diabetes (although we had no tests to substantiate this as he would not see a doctor). He said he had been lucky so far. In one consultation he was given an understanding of what he was buying as far as health risks and nutrition were concerned, guidance as to the best quality of food he could afford, and very importantly, the balance of foods he needed each day to ensure he had the energy he wanted and needed for healing and repair. He was encouraged to juice to help with nutritional saturation, and limited supplements were suggested just to give his body some short-term help.

He informed me he was going away for a two-week holiday but he would start to make the changes when he got back. Six weeks later I spoke with him (four weeks into his change of lifestyle) and this is what he had to say in his own words (permission received).

18 July, 2012

I met Jasmine while undertaking work at her home with my business.

She noticed I walked with a bit of a limp, and I informed her of past ligament damage to my knees.

And that I was worried about a probable circulation problem, having numbness in my feet.

I arranged a consultation with Jasmine, where we discussed my diet and the effects foods and additives were having on my body.

After having learnt to read labels on food, and changing my diet to her recommendations, I am amazed by the results.

My numbness has disappeared, I feel 300 per cent better in myself, and my energy levels and attention to work has completely turned around. As an added bonus, although not considering myself on a diet as such, just changing my eating patterns and the food I eat, I have lost 10kg in just over a month.

An employee of mine also visited Jasmine, and as a result, his doctor cannot believe the change in his blood pressure, cholesterol levels and liver functions.

I cannot recommend Jasmine's services enough, and do so to all my friends.

If you value your health, want to feel better, and look better, please give her a visit.

Thank you Jasmine, I really appreciate your help, and your non-pushy, friendly manner, and the genuine interest you take in me.

Regards Steve

(Permission given to print)

Some people will come and see me with specific problems like high cholesterol, arthritis, asthma, weight problems, digestive disorders and more serious chronic and auto immune diseases, but as the body is treated as a whole, starting with eating the right foods, they are surprised when other aches and pains, and health issues disappear. They also lose weight as their body rebalances and starts to heal and they have more energy. Often the whole family benefits from the changes too. Others want to prevent health problems and chronic disease but don't know how to go about it.

Step by step I am going to guide you through how you can change your approach to eating. I will give you practical knowledge to enable you to make a permanent change both to improve your health and to protect you from sickness.

SO LET'S STEP FORWARD TO A HEALTHY LIFE

WHAT DOES OUR BODY NEED FOR GOOD HEALTH?

- Good food
- Fresh living water
- Sunshine
- Fresh air
- Exercise
- A good laugh!

WE SHOULD EAT TO LIVE – NOT LIVE TO EAT

- Good food means fresh nutritious wholefood.
- Fresh living water means no fluoride, no chlorine, no chemicals.
- Sunshine means at least half an hour at midday exposing the torso, both sides, to the healing rays of the sun to enable us to absorb vitamin D which protects us from cancer and other diseases.
- Fresh air means to escape if we can into our gardens, or the beach, or the mountains, back to nature where the air is cleaner and more healing.
- Exercise, such as a good walk half an hour morning and night is a good start.
- A good laugh. Not only is laughter healing, a lighter outlook rather than a heavy one which is so prevalent in today's society is far better for your wellbeing. Be positive!

CHAPTER 2

STEP 1
UNDERSTAND WHAT YOU ARE EATING

One of the first things I teach people is to look very closely at what they are buying to put into their mouth. I ask them to consider, if I eat or drink this, will it serve my body well or might it harm me?

ADDITIVES

It is very important to understand that food additives can be cumulative (I believe they all are and I don't believe in safe additives and I will tell you why later). You see, we were first led to believe that the small amounts we ate in food, the body would be able to eliminate them. But there are now some 3000 food additives, and each product we buy can contain several. We are no longer eating just a few!

If there is only one thing you learn from this book it would be for you to understand the detrimental effects of food additives and avoid them ALL. You and your family will benefit tremendously.

JASMINE MAKINGS

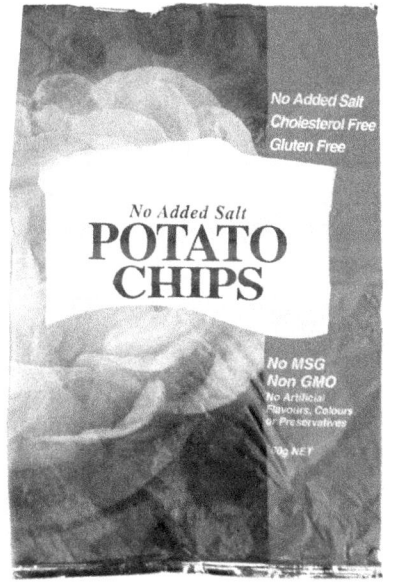

Take a look at this product bought from the health section of a supermarket. (Name blocked out for obvious reasons.) It looks good, no added salt, cholesterol free, gluten free, no MSG, no GMO, no artificial flavours, colours or preservatives. What could possibly be wrong with this? Well if you turn over the packet and find the tiny little word 'ingredients' you would see that the ingredients are; potatoes, palm oil (antioxidants 319, 330). If you check out what in fact 319 is you would find that it is tert-butylhydroquinone (contains a petroleum derivative, often used with BHA and BHT, banned in some countries). Its 'potential sides effects are "moderately toxic by ingestion, birth defects, tinnitus, allergic contact dermatitis, may be carcinogenic and mutagenic. It is also used in the production of suntan lotion, hair colouring and cosmetics.

Natural oils that are organic and cold-pressed have short shelf lives, so they tend not to be used in commercial cooking and are expensive. Therefore the cheaper refined vegetable oils – which contain some of the worst food additives 310, 319 and 320 which have been linked to cancer and other serious side effects – are more commonly used.

The additive 319, which is petroleum based and should be avoided, has been linked to cancer, birth defects, can cause nausea, vomiting, delirium, collapse and dermatitis. Supposedly, an acceptable Daily Intake is Up to 0.02mg/kg body weight. A dose of 5g is considered fatal. Products which may contain this are dairy blend edible fats and oils, margarine, dripping, salad dressing, lipsticks.

Most if not all food additives come out of chemical factories. Examples are –

Number	Side effects	Used for	Also used for
260 (regarded as Safe)	skin irritation, hives, cancer in rats	fruit wine, mead veg wine foods for infants	animal feeds, hair dyes hand lotions, cigarettes adhesives

And even so called 'natural' ones also regarded as safe such as –

Number	Side effects	Used for	Also used for
412 (From seeds of a tree)	possible abdominal cramps and obstruction, flatulence, nausea, diarrhoea	infant formula products, foods for infants	binding tablets, cosmetics, slimming aids (caution advised)

Many of the preservatives (and there are a lot), added to processed food, meat products in our butcher shops, such as cured meats, sausages, marinated meats, are 'asthma triggers'.

Example

| 211 | asthma, urticaria, contact Dermatitis, hay fever, Mouth and skin irritation, | jams, spreads, glace cherries, icings ... | toothpaste, eye creams, cosmetics, medical diagnostic aid for liver function |

IMPORTANT: In Australia there is also a 5% loophole in the law regarding food labelling. This hole in the legislation means that manufacturers do not have to list some ingredients in a product. This can be regardless of how toxic it is to human health. Please check such loopholes in your country of residence.

For example, some of the antioxidants (such as 310, 319 or 320) are banned in other countries and are associated with adverse health effects. But these additives are not listed on labels if the amount in the product is less than 5% of its total weight. Manufacturers can list compound ingredients and not list what is in those ingredients if they make up less than 5% of the final product. These ingredients often contain suspect antioxidants, colours and preservatives.

There are no Warnings on food labels of possible adverse effects of additives either. For example many preservatives, especially sulphites and nitrates, are well known asthma triggers and yet are widely used in fresh and processed foods with no warnings to asthmatics.

There are also many additives that are specifically banned in foods intended for infants and young children because of their proven adverse health impacts. And whilst they may be kept out of foods such as infant formula and baby food, they can be widely used in other products eaten by children, especially snacks like chips, crackers, savouries etc.

The potential short and long-term side effects and damage which can be attributed to food additives is enormous. You will not find any warnings on labels, so again I ask you to study the ingredients of everything you buy, and establish exactly what it is and what it can cause before you put it in your mouth.

Case Study – Asthma

Another case was a 22-year-old young woman (whose father was a medical doctor). She had asthma from childhood. As always I try to encourage clients to avoid ALL additives – as I believe sooner or later they are likely to cause health problems – rather than just removing specific symptom-related additives as in asthma. This young lady apparently was having about three bad attacks a week but immediately on removing all additives from her diet her attacks stopped. Three months later, which was when I last saw her, she hadn't had any attacks. This young lady's asthma had been severe, not only did she carry inhalers but breathing apparatus as well. We were again in touch after about six years and still she was having no attacks. By computer messaging she informed me:

> *"I'm very slim now, no chocolates any more as I used to eat, I eat lots of vegetables, fish and fruits – I must be grateful for you – I've never had any more problems with asthma, I think it is because I go jogging every day and also the food change." Name withheld*

It is quite common knowledge that certain food additives are attributed to behavioural problems in children and not only children.

Case study - Insomnia & hallucinations, concentration & hyperactivity

A few years ago, back in England, I knocked on the door of a neighbour who promptly told me that he and his wife had had a really bad night. He said they hadn't slept all night, they even felt they had been hallucinating. I asked what they had had for their evening meal and he said nothing that they hadn't eaten before. What about drink I asked? We only had a bottle of flavoured water he said, but we haven't had it before. I asked him if I could see the bottle. It was spring water with elderflower and the only other added ingredient was a preservative. I am sorry it was so long ago I don't remember which one but I remember the side effects very clearly which were insomnia and hallucinations. My neighbour was grateful to at least know what had caused their very disturbing night and said they would not be buying that product again!

Colourings are a particular problem when it comes to behaviour, and at last count I understand there are 80,000 children in Australia (reported cases), with behavioural issues, now branded as a disease known as ADHD.

Example

Number	Side effects	Used for	Also used for
102	Asthma, urticaria, dermatitis, headache, hay fever, concentration difficulties, depression, skin rash learning difficulties, behavioural problems, swelling of lips and tongue,	beverages and processed foods	cosmetics, wool and silk dye, drugs

I would say all colours, which are usually numbered in the hundreds, have the same or similar side effects. So imagine how many different additives are in a packet of different coloured sweets for example! There are so many of these, in so much of our food and drinks, and the above side effects are typical of them.

Testimonial

In recent years I had a consultation with a young mother (who coincidentally worked in the medical profession). One of her children, an eight-year-old girl, had been having behavioural problems for a while, so much so the whole family was affected and the mother was very distressed. The only course of action on offer was to give the child the drug Ritalin and she knew full well what these drugs were and did not want to go that route. When I offered her 'another way' she was extremely willing to do whatever it took. Our second meeting was at her home (not my normal practice but it was an exception) and I spent time with the mother, going through her pantry and teaching her how to read food labels so she could fully understand what she was buying. I later learned as soon as I had left, she emptied the pantry and put all the food in the refuse bin and went out to shop for fresh food before her children came home from school. This is what I call a sweep clean – for some people it is too overwhelming and they have to make changes step by step. This is the testimonial from the lady in question.

> *I consider myself to be very fortunate to have been introduced to Jasmine at a time when we were really struggling to cope with our 8 year old daughter's behaviour. It would be fair to say we were at a loss as to what to do, nothing we had tried thus far had had any impact on her aggressive sometimes violent outbursts. She had difficulty concentrating for any length of time, was at times agitated, was extremely difficult to settle at night and suffered from chronic constipation. When I confided my distress at all of this and my concerns for our daughter's future health I was instantly reassured that we would be able to make changes in our diet that would benefit her.*
>
> *Jasmine came to our home and spent a lot of time explaining and sharing her knowledge on food labelling and the adverse effects of the chemicals in our foods. Jasmine made recommendations, which have been simple to implement but that have had a major impact on our whole family.*
>
> *Our daughter is now calmer, sleeps better, goes to the toilet regularly, is achieving consistently at school and is a pleasant, confident, happy little girl.*
>
> *Our whole family has benefited from the changes we have made and I am now confident that I am making healthy, informed choices for my family based on Jasmines advice. Rebecca – Jan., 2012. (permission to print)*

How many children are taking medical drugs for this unnecessarily?

Let's look at a few more of these additives to help you fully realise just how harmful they can be –

Number	Side effects	Used for	Also used for
220	Asthma, broncho spasm, hypotension, bronchitis, bronchoconstriction, destroys vitamins A and B1	jams, spreads dried fruits and veg, desiccated coconut biscuits, cakes, pastries	glue, disinfectant in breweries and food factories
621 MSG	Bronchospasm, heart palpitations abdominal discomfort, irritability fibromyalgia, nausea, depression headache, migraine, asthma, blurred vision, vertigo, sight impairment, teratogenic,	flavour enhancer found in soups, soy sauce, flavourings for meats and chicken and natural flavouring	*see below

*Also used for: soap, cosmetics, shampoo, hair conditioner and MOST LIVE VIRUS VACCINES

Please also note that many other names are being used for this additive as people become more aware of its dangers.

SAFE ADDITIVES?

As I said earlier I do not believe in safe additives simply because what is believed today can change tomorrow. Let me give you an example. Twenty-five years ago when my dear friend gave me a little book about E numbers (which I still have although in tatters with use) this is what it stated regarding additive 160b.

Number	Side effects	Used for	Also used for
In 1980s – **160b** as below (A natural extract from a tree)	NO KNOWN SIDE EFFECTS	as below	as below
And currently - **160b**	May cause irritability, head banging in children, urticarial and pruritis from skin contact still undergoing testing!	flavoured milk, ice-cream noodles, cakes, pastries pasta, milk products	fabric dye and varnish, body paints, soaps

NB – SAFETY & TESTING

It is very important to note that additives are usually tested on animals and are usually tested as a single component, and the so called 'safety' level is derived at a point where an animal is adversely affected. What are not tested are combinations and effects of these additives when put together. So whilst one additive in itself may not have obvious side effects immediately, together they can be very harmful indeed. I also repeat that additives are accumulative in the body, just as sodium fluoride is in our water, and can build up to dangerous harmful levels causing long-term health problems.

WHAT DO I BUY INSTEAD?

Of course I would not encourage anyone to buy processed 'dead' foods in the first instance but I appreciate we all have to lean on things in packets etc. occasionally. Therefore, once you understand how to read labels it will soon become clear to you that anything with numbers or chemical sounding names are to be avoided. You will find products without these additives; they used to be few but as demand grows supermarkets and mainly health stores are now stocking more. But please do not be tempted to buy because of what the marketing says on the front of the packet – this is to persuade you to buy it. You will find the truth of the ingredients, probably in very small print somewhere else on the packet. Look for the word 'ingredients' and see what it contains before you purchase. However, please keep such foods to a minimum even if you find those with ingredients not as 'harmful as the rest' because they do not nourish you and eating any amount of these just diminishes your appetite for the real food.

You know if you make a cake or a biscuit it would contain perhaps flour, butter, sugar, eggs, so if the packet lists ten, twenty ingredients, you know there is something wrong. Beware also of trick names such as natural flavour, extracts such as malt or yeast as many manufactures are now trying to camouflage additive names because people are getting wise to their dangers.

READING YOUR LABELS AND UNDERSTANDING WHAT YOU ARE BUYING TO CONSUME IS PROBABLY THE MOST IMPORTANT FIRST STEP YOU CAN TAKE.

I find that once people realise they are eating chemicals which are also in shampoos, creams, detergents etc. they no longer want to buy them. Almost automatically they become more aware of the importance of considering what they put in their mouth! When you start to realise this and no longer buy this type of food, you will automatically lean towards 'fresher' food.

As a guide there are pocket sized books on the market which explain the numbers, their names and their side effects, but once you get used to checking labels you will not need a reference book, and once you realise what is in these products, and the side effects, you won't want to buy them, hopefully.

Why not try the local markets where often people make 'homemade' food to sell and you can ask them what the ingredients are!

MISLEADING LABELLING REGARDING NUTRITION.

When the Western world became concerned about 'fats' triggered I believe by such as the BSA crisis in cattle and salmonella fears in eggs, the food industry were alerted to change their approach (and packaging) or lose business. They jumped on board and started producing hundreds of 'low fat' products to cater for those who were looking to eat healthier. What we trusting innocents didn't realise that in place of the fats, they just added more sugar for flavour. This in turn has created over-consumption of sugars and syrups and has no doubt hugely contributed not only to the obesity crisis but young people with diseases such as cancer, diabetes, arthritis and lupus. We all trusted yet again that what is on the shelves for sale must be okay or it would not be allowed to be there.

Therefore, it is very important not only to check the 'ingredient labels' but the nutritional content too in respect of sugar, salts and carbs. Personally, having looked into the labelling of foods, the information cannot be totally relied upon as correct so I am extremely careful about the few things I do buy with labels on them. I also repeat, anything in packets, bottles, cartons, even frozen has little or no nutrition after all the processing, additives etc. What is the point in putting it into your body anyway!

COMMENTS

I think everyone these days is aware of the dangers of fast food/junk food; it's been in the media long enough because of the obesity epidemic! I don't have to convince people who choose to eat these that they are eating the wrong thing and they know it.

The difficult ones to convince are the ones who perhaps shop at the supermarket for almost everything, say they don't eat fast foods and tell me they cook! Well guess what, many years ago I was a mum who cooked and shopped at the supermarket for most things, but I was horrified to find many additives in the food I considered 'fresh', and good for my family, were not what I thought they were. For example cheeses, fruit yogurts, chicken fillets, bread. I did not consider these foods junk but when I looked at the ingredients and checked with my little book I realised I was very much mistaken. Firstly, I felt extremely guilty that I had been feeding my loved ones on food with additives (even though it was fresh food) and then I was very angry and I felt misled. I had trusted the food industry, the authorities, the people who do all the checks on what is fit to eat and what is not and I had wrongly assumed that if they are on the supermarket shelf they must be safe. And of course in those days I was not aware of all the drugs being fed to animals and the way they were being farmed. Nowadays, on the few occasions I buy meat of any kind I would ensure it was organic.

I also realised that the ones responsible for this misconception – let's be kind and say through ignorance – would not be open to my complaints. I decided then, if anyone could make a difference it is the consumer. If the consumer is aware and does not buy such products the supermarkets will be left with them on their shelves and that will cost them money, and likewise their suppliers. Perhaps then they will listen. We have seen this happening already as consumers are becoming more aware.

So about thirty years ago I started talking, teaching, spreading the word and working with individuals. Later this developed into group workshops, speaking at coffee mornings and seminars. People don't need to suffer the way they do as so many ailments and illness are avoidable but a lot of people can't seem to accept that simply changing what they eat can make them better! If only they knew that it is what they eat that probably caused their health problems in the first place.

I did once write to HRH Prince Charles about the danger of additives. My husband and I had been privileged to visit Highgrove. We spent the whole morning on the Prince's organic farm. It was wonderful and amazing. Why did we ever drift from this healthy way of farming? All the organic produce was boxed and sold in the surrounding villages. I was envious as the part of England where we lived was very much supermarket and imported foods and very limited organic. After lunch our afternoon was a tour of the beautiful gardens of Highgrove, a natural meadow being my favourite. I have a lot of respect and admiration for HRH, what he has achieved on his farm at Highgrove. I urge everyone to read his book *Harmony*. Prince Charles has a love of nature and of this planet which provides for us, and he has the knowledge of how to protect it. We should listen to him!

OTHER FOODS (AND DRINKS) WHICH ARE HARMFUL TO OUR HEALTH

GENETICALLY MODIFIED FOOD (GMO)

I thought things could not get any worse in respect of the food industry and our water quality after the implementation of sodium fluoride around the world (which thankfully is now being banned in many countries) and that nothing could shock me – but I was mistaken.

It is very important to be aware and to avoid genetically modified food. Not only is this food detrimental to health, it is also detrimental to farming and to nature and to the future of food, and worse still the future of our planet. It is one of the scariest things that has happened in my lifetime. Its effects on the body are not being fully revealed and I urge you to keep well away from these foods and to fully investigate the full implications connected with this practice.

My understanding is that these foods are not tested by independent bodies but manufacturers are trusted to do their own testing. Ingredients used cause the stomachs of bugs and insects to split when they eat them, while allergies have increased dramatically in countries eating GMO. Some doctors are advising patients not to eat them. There have been warnings that GMO foods may create allergies, poisons, new diseases. Land once contaminated with these crops will be very difficult to restore, if ever, and of course natural germination is interfered with if not halted forever.

I was asked recently 'well don't people have a choice as to what food they buy', my answer was, 'yes, but not usually an informed choice'! Hopefully, by the time you have read this book you will be very informed. For further information on this subject I would refer you to GMO DANGERS by Mr Jeffrey Smith who is an international bestselling author and filmmaker and is the leading spokesperson on the health dangers of GMO foods.

This is really serious and I hope this information will stir you into researching fully for yourself if you are tempted to eat this food! If you value your health and that of future generations don't buy this food. It is not natural!

DRINKS/FLUIDS

WATER

SODIUM FLUORIDE is another additive which has serious side effects. This is a registered poison. Look for yourself; you don't have to take my word for it. We are led to believe that such and such an amount will help teeth and will not harm our body. Even if there is any truth in this belief, it still does not justify medicating and subjecting the masses to the potential serious long-term side effects of this toxic waste. The authorities' argument that a small controlled amount will not harm is misleading, and the worst of it is that there is no way of knowing how much each individual has. As one person may drink one glass of tap water a day someone else may be drinking a couple of litres. Each individual will bathe in fluoridated water which will be absorbed through their skin into their bloodstream and into each organ! Their food and other drinks will be made, washed, cooked in fluoridated water, and their vegetables may have been watered with it when growing. They may clean their teeth with fluoridated toothpaste, which by the way if you read the label it will tell you it's poison and not to swallow it. How do you stop young children from doing that, and it is cumulative and very harmful to health. The fact is that it is raw toxic waste from aluminium and fertiliser plants, neurotoxic and has many adverse health effects proven throughout the world.

One must ask why with so much information and proof available and with so many side effects and potential dangers to our health, did authorities around the world put this in water supplies under the pretext of one possible but disputable health benefit! Thankfully in recent years most of Europe has banned it, the European Law courts made a ruling it is in fact a medication and of course it is against human rights to mass medicate. Few countries continue to use it in spite of the public outcry! One has to ask the question why some authorities still insist on polluting our water with this unnecessary poison?

We have reverse osmosis in our kitchen, one single tap which we use for washing and cooking all of our food and for drinking water. We only use tap water for cleaning; and unfortunately showering (with filters). Our herbs and vegetables are watered with rainwater. Reverse osmosis is far from perfect but it isn't toxic. When you fully understand the dangers of sodium fluoride I hope you make your stand against its use, enforced use at that!

Ordinary filters will not remove fluoride from our tap water, only reverse osmosis which can be quite expensive. There are local companies who offer reverse osmosis installation. The downside is that it takes everything out of the water so you need to ensure minerals are put back in but even then it is not the same as 'living water'.

DEHYDRATION

Our body is made up of over 70 per cent water and we need to keep our levels topped up. Dehydration in itself can be very detrimental to health and cause many symptoms and likewise many symptoms will disappear when we make the effort to drink more water and alkaline drinks. Apart from being needed for all bodily functions, looking at the practical side, it helps flush out toxins from our body via our skin and kidneys. Imagine your kitchen sink clogged up with waste and you don't run the tap to help it flush out, or worse still the toilet!

Therefore, the quality of the water we drink is very important whether by the glass or making herb teas, juices etc.

A few years ago a neighbour asked if I could help her very young daughter who was constantly getting migraines. It seemed to always happen at school following sport activities. Dehydration is a big contributor to migraines (as well as many other health problems). People tend to drink water during and after sport or physical exertion, but the damage can already be done. If the body is dehydrated to start with, it becomes more so during such exertion therefore it is important to drink before exertion as well as during and after. A few grains of natural mineral/rock salt added will help tremendously.

TEA

Tea is acid, and with milk affects digestion so keep it to a minimum.

COFFEE

Coffee is also acid and can adversely affect digestion if made with milk. It is better to drink it black. Instant coffees are processed and therefore not natural. Coffee also prevents absorption of iron! However, natural black coffee can be very helpful early morning to help clean out the intestines! It is also used widely in coffee enemas to help the body detoxify.

Tea and coffee as well as being acidic (acid/alkaline balance will be explained a little later), they are also very dehydrating. So if you are a regular tea or coffee drinker, you will need to increase your water intake to compensate and counteract the dehydrating effects. Ideally, try to reduce intake to one cup a day.

Juices Processed

Juices in bottles, packets and tins are processed in some way regardless of what it says on the label regarding 100 per cent natural or no added ingredients etc. The first problem is that the juice is not always the whole fruit and does not contain the fibre, often it is reconstituted and not in its natural state. Fruit juices can be high in natural sugars, but many processed juices may also have added sugar and may also have preservatives, colours and flavours added.

ALCOHOL

Like tea and coffee, alcohol is acid and very dehydrating, as well as all the other known dangers to health and wellbeing. The same applies to limiting such drinking and increasing other alkaline drinks which will help dilute and rebalance.

RECOMMENDED FLUIDS

Juices HOME MADE

A fruit is made up of the skin, the pith, the flesh and seeds. This is whole fruit – in a whole food; nature gives us a combination of complementary vitamins and minerals. If we extract only the juice, it is no longer complete and natural and we no longer receive the full benefit of the rest of the fruit. If you have a cold pressed kind of juicer, which extracts the juice and leaves the fibre behind, you can use the waste fibre in soups or dehydrate and sprinkle on salads, muesli, etc. There are also juicers available where, in most cases, they will juice beautifully most skins, seeds and core i.e. the whole fruit for our benefit.

One of the beauties of juicing is that it is a wonderful way of getting vital nutrients into your body, and as a liquid, even people with poor appetite or sick people can manage to drink juices. Juicing is widely used in natural and integrative clinics around the world in their programmes of treating people to improve their health.

A client of mine (mentioned at the beginning of the book) had several major health problems and was declining rapidly. Apart from having had a heart attack in recent years and a stent inserted into an artery (obviously indicating inflammation of the arteries and high cholesterol), she was also diabetic, had stage 4 kidney failure and pancreatitis, which entailed frequent bouts in hospital as a result of 'eating'; and dialysis was looming. Although we started this lady on a high-nutrient liquid diet, it had to be done cautiously as the kidneys couldn't handle a lot of fluids. This was a serious situation indeed, and juicing with high nutrients was a life saver until such time as we could start to build up other foods, albeit cautiously. Within months we achieved low cholesterol, stabilised blood sugar, stabilised the kidneys, and settled attacks of pancreatitis and no hospital admissions. The lady in question has her life back, not spent sleeping at home or in hospital, she has more energy and a better quality of life. Of course we are hoping to continue to improve her health, but the emphasis here is on the support and importance of juicing. Not just to sustain life in this instance but to give ourselves the amount of nutrients we cannot always manage to eat in our modern busy world.

HERB TEAS

Can be very therapeutic and medicinal and often I ask clients either to drink these instead of other teas/coffees etc., and in some case ask them to drink specific herbal teas to help the body such as:

Peppermint tea can sooth the digestive system.

Sage and yarrow teas help clean the kidneys. Sage helps strengthen bones, and Yarrow is good to help inflammation and women's menstrual problems.

Chamomile is calming for the nerves, soothing to the digestive system.

Some years ago I recommended a nursing mum to drink chamomile tea three times a day. She was stressed; the baby was always crying, no doubt sensing the mum's stress and getting colic too. The baby benefited from the chamomile through the mum's breast milk and both became very calm and content and slept better. I would even give babies a very mild chamomile in aired water, i.e. one dip of an organic chamomile teabag which would have the same effect.

FILERED WATER

Drink the best quality filtered water you can afford. Reverse osmosis was mentioned previously. Any kind of home filter system is better than nothing and there is also good mineral water available but ensure it is bottled in glass and not plastic.

SUMMARY OF STEP 1

1. Read your ingredient labels before buying anything to eat or drink.

2. Don't eat or drink anything which contains additives.

3. Avoid all junk food and processed foods and each more fresh.

4. Fresh local produce is the most nutritious.

5. Don't buy GMO foods.

Fluids

1. Drink plenty of filtered water – 2 litres a day is the norm for an average person.

2. Drink herb teas.

3. Drink home-made fruit and vegetable juices.

4. Try to keep to one tea/coffee per day.

CHAPTER 3

STEP 2
WHAT WE SHOULD AND SHOULD NOT EAT

It is important to buy the best quality local fresh produce we can. It is surprising how much we spend on clothes, cars and holidays, but when it comes to the most important thing we need for good health we don't always buy the best quality!

Local fresh is best. We have a good permaculture vegetable and herb garden at home but I shop once a week at the local organic market for vegetables, greens, fruit, salads, eggs and milk. If I run out in the course of the week I shop at a local organic store or a good quality fruit and veg market ensuring that I buy Australian produce only. This is the best food I can buy for my family as far as nutrition is concerned but also avoids all the chemicals used in agriculture these days. In addition I am supporting local farmers to keep up their good work for our benefit and that of future generations.

I shop at the local supermarket once every few months for toilet rolls etc!

Other organic produce such as whole flour, cider vinegar, oats, lentils, beans, spices, dried fruits, nuts, oils, I buy wholesale.

I don't actually spend much time shopping at all which suits me very much and means I can use my time for other important things. I am surprised at the number of people who are 'always popping to the shop' for something for dinner! Time, petrol, and what price and quality of produce can they buy?

We now have our own vegetable and herb garden made for us by Gold Coast Permaculture. In this photograph it is ready for this season's planting but you can see that the soil has been built up to form the garden. This is because this piece of garden was all gravel and we could not plant anything. You can even have vegetable boxes placed in areas of unusable garden or patios.

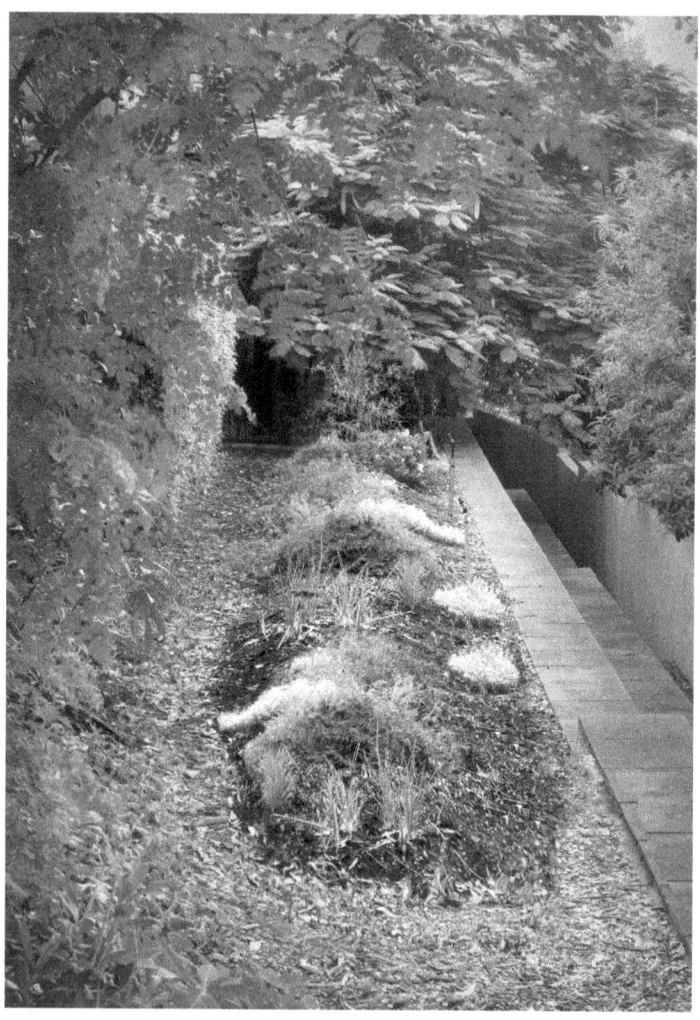

Consequently our meals and snacks are fresh, nutritious and simple. I love eating good tasty food but I don't like spending a lot of time in the kitchen. Therefore, also consider some raw food which can be simply delicious, requires little preparation and no sweating over hot stoves in the summer. There are many simple recipes online these days so we won't go into this subject now but try it. Bear in mind that raw foods (salads & juicing for example) don't have nutrients destroyed with cooking so they can contain a lot of vitamins, minerals and enzymes which the body needs to repair, for its fuel and digestion. Juices are a lot easier to digest than solids, so bear this in mind when you are healing.

One hundred per cent PLANT based diets are not unusual to promote healing the body and getting the immune system working properly. Integrated doctors, 'natural clinics' and healing centres around the world use this philosophy successfully. Take a look at the documentary video 'raw in 30 days' and see how Gabriel Cousens treats several long standing insulin dependent diabetics using this principle to reverse their disease in 30 days! Many will probably focus on Dr Gerson's philosophy of detoxification and nutritional saturation, using, in particular, a lot of juicing. As an example, at the Gerson Institute, according to their book *Healing the Gerson Way*, a patient would take a specific juice every hour over a 12-hour period, consuming something like 8kg (17lbs) of vegetables and 5.5kg (12lbs) of fruit. This is nutritional saturation. We couldn't possibly eat those amounts each day. That is in addition to three specific meals and of course a lot of detoxification which is essential in this work.

My focus with any client is always without fail is to encourage them to avoid all processed and inflammatory foods and to eat a lot more fresh food, including juicing. The health benefits become very clear in a very short time.

A recent young client, diagnosed with Lupus was already having symptoms of joint pain (rheumatoid arthritis), kidney problems, skin problems and lacking energy. In less than two weeks his large, patchy red skin had dried up, his joint pain had gone and he was very happy with the extra energy. It is very early days at this point but I am confident we will see much improved results in the coming months if he perseveres.

I was asked recently - what is typical day's eating plan for me – just to give a picture of life without additives and processed foods.

An example of how to eat more living food daily.

		Alternative suggestions
BREAKFAST	Fresh fruits and juice (homemade)	with sheeps yogurt
	Poached eggs or omelette with perhaps, spinach, and tomato	Organic porridge oats chia seeds and banana
	Or avocado chopped and sprinkled with lots of lemon juice, olive oil, and roasted seeds	
11'S	Smoothie made with nut milk, fruits,	Pineapple, melon, banana
	You can add a raw egg yolk and one tsp raw honey	
	Chia seeds or organic fruit wheat free toast	Spinach or kale, apple, berries
	Juices with seasonable fruit adding nuts and chia seeds	
LUNCH	Salad of green leaves, avocado, celery, Fetta cheese, apple, tomato, lemon juice	or boiled eggs nut cheese/hummus/flax
	In cooler weather I make lots of homemade soups	
SNACK	Healthy homemade snacks like chocolate crunch	
	Or a protein ball, crackers with nut pastes	
DINNER	Steamed vegetables with a lentil dish or brown rice	
	Or vegetable casserole with chickpeas or lentils	Lamb or organic chicken

COMMENTS: Chia seeds, lentils, chickpeas, nut cheeses and a lot of vegetables, particularly greens, all contain alternative protein to animal protein/meats. We eat lots of fruit and vegetables every day not just in meals but in lots of juicing too.

Don't forget to use herbs and spices and experiment, including using them in juices, salads, soups and sauces. They are very nutritious and medicinal.

And our body likes change, variety, so don't have the same meals all the time.

My herb garden

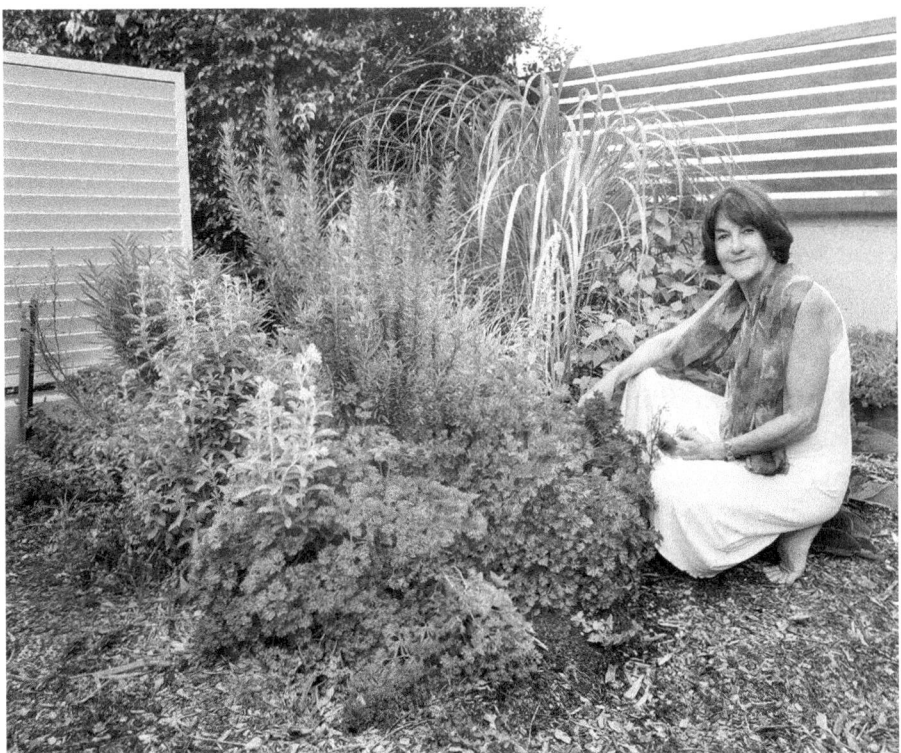

If you do not have room for a herb garden, a pot of fresh herbs on your kitchen worktop would encourage you to pick them and include them in meal and drink preparation.

FLUIDS

I make 1-2 litres of juice in the morning so we can drink throughout the day. Then it is one job and one lot of cleaning. We also drink various herb teas, such as liquorice, lemon grass, and also filtered and spring water etc.

Nut Milks. Whilst these can be bought in packets from the supermarket and health stores, read labels as they could contain other things, mainly preservatives. It is so easy to make your own if you have a good blender and you can concoct a mixture to contribute to the different nutrients you need.

The one I make mostly because it is so flexible is cashew nut milk. (One cup of cashew nuts to two cups of filtered water, blended). It is white and creamy and I don't have to soak the nuts overnight. I stir this into our porridge which I have made with water and add the nut milk after cooking. Almond milk is also very good.

Sometimes I add a few sunflower and sesame seeds to my cashew nut milk too which are highly nutritious. This is good to drink on its own too, perhaps with a little vanilla essence or honey.

More examples of smoothies/juices.

- Frozen mixed berries (preservative free) banana, apple, fresh mint, green leaves and/or fresh herbs
- Or, watermelon, pineapple, kale or spinach, ice cubes
- Or, carrot, celery, apple, with or without green leaves. I add lots of fresh herbs too.

For a protein drink I use a handful of almonds and often add super foods like chia seeds, a banana, berries and 1-2 raw organic egg yolks and a little raw honey (to kill any bacteria).

It is good to add dark leafy greens for the minerals, particularly magnesium, iron and calcium, and herbs for the minerals and their medicinal qualities.

If we feel we need a cleanse or are dehydrated I would make a couple of litres of pure watermelon juice with the fibre, pop it in the fridge and drink throughout the day on an empty stomach.

SALADS

In early marriage my husband used to call salad rabbit food and would not eat it – it wasn't filling enough for men. Today he embraces all the salads I make. Instead of just the basic lettuce and tomato we used to have as children, I include dried fruits, fresh fruits, seeds and nuts, cheeses, lots of lemon juice and olive oil. Our salads are a filling, nutritious meal which satisfies even my husband's stomach!

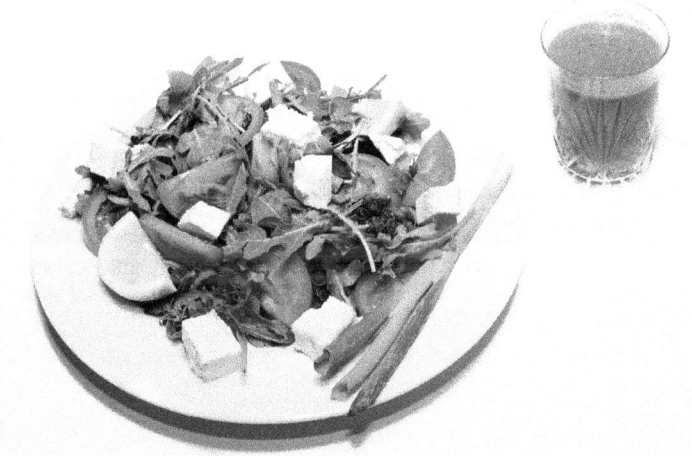

Pear salad with goat's cheese – and a healthy blueberry smoothie!

I am often asked what I do if I want to eat out. First of all I am very particular as to where I eat out, and when I do I speak with the chef/staff as to where the food comes from and what they use for such things as oils and dressings. Otherwise I stick with salads, steamed vegetables and plain chicken or omelette. I don't have any foods which are mixed together like a risotto or bolognaise unless I am absolutely sure it only contains fresh food, spices, herbs and no processed food or stock cubes of any kind. If when you ask about ingredients just mention you have reactions to additives so it is important that you know what's in the dish, you are then more likely to receive more co-operation.

I do have some special places which I trust implicitly!

I am reminded of a local bistro opening in one of the local villages in England and they advertised home-made soup and sandwich for lunch. One day my husband and I decided to give it a try. I first asked the waiter what the soup was and if in fact it was home made. Yes! As it was tomato soup on that day I asked if any tomato paste was used out of a tube (as this can contain preservatives and flavours). No he insisted it was all home-made and off he went to the kitchen. He then walked out with a large tin in one hand and a packet in the other. These were the ingredients of the 'home-made' soup. They mix stuff from the tin and the packet and mix together with water and heat it. So that was their version of home made. Another slogan is home cooked (that doesn't mean home-made by the way). PS I didn't order it!

ACID/ALKALINE BALANCE

The importance of eating an 80/20 diet of alkaline foods/acid foods cannot go unmentioned.

The Western diet of excessive processed carbohydrates, sugars and unhealthy fats has contributed to acid bodies and poor health. Acid bodies are open to every sniffle, cough, virus, infection, disease and cancer prevalent in society today.

Dr Otto Warburg was awarded two Nobel prizes in the mid 1900s for his work on the cause and cure of cancer. His statement that 'no disease can survive in an alkalised environment' should be encouragement enough to ensure your body is in fact an alkaline environment if you desire wellbeing.

There is no doubt that acidity/acidosis is the prime cause of disease and we need to do everything we can to ensure our body is not subject to this condition. It is not easy with the 'Western style diet' which is principally acid, and our toxic environment both sometimes in the home and outside exposes us to more and more acid waste. When acid waste accumulates in our body we are exposed to disease of all kinds. The foundation of alkalinity must start with the diet, food and drink. Also very important to ensure we eliminate the acid waste. It is easy to print a list of the alkaline/acid foods off the internet which will give you every category of food, oils, grains, plants, herbs as a quick guide. Alkaline foods tend to be more fresh foods, and processed foods acid, but check them out to be sure.

ELIMINATION

We cannot go any further without mentioning the importance of an efficient elimination system. Of course our elimination system consists of our skin, (often skin problems can be attributed to toxins in the body trying to get out), our lungs, our kidney, liver, bowels etc.

We can eat the best diet in the world but if our body doesn't eliminate properly and regularly then all that good stuff can become toxic waste and end up in our blood stream. If you watch a newborn babe, it has a bowel movement after every feed. We should empty our bowels three times a day if our bowels are functioning at maximum efficiency. You have heard of the saying I am sure that death begins in the bowel, now you know why.

Therefore, the basis of good elimination is of course a good diet, but we need lots of fibre in the diet. (I was listening to a documentary recently that attributed a high-fibre diet to reducing and re-balancing blood sugar and a host of other health benefits too). I have mentioned natural remedies later in the book to help with constipation, but you need to take a long-term view, not a quick fix to ensure bowel efficiency. I would highly recommend colonic hydrotherapy, preferably the treatments where the therapist sits with you and who can make several adjustments during the course of the treatment for your comfort. My belief is that everyone should consider this 'clean out' as the build-up in our tubes over many years, and in some cases many decades, can amount to several kilos of hardened waste. Not only is this highly toxic, but it also prevents the proper absorption of nutrients, so unless this is removed all that good food may not be absorbing properly into your system.

Some years ago when I was doing a series of workshops which embraced teaching about food/health/dangers of additives etc., I presented a specific session on the harmful effects of constipation. At the end of the workshop a lady approach me and burst into tears. She pointed to her abdomen which was enlarged, swollen and hard. She said she felt ghastly and hadn't been to the bathroom for a few days and she was distressed and didn't know what to do as nothing so far had worked. Naturally, I explained the necessity to ensure a balanced diet to correct the problem, but as an 'emergency remedy' I asked her to take one teaspoon of organic castor oil as soon as she got home, to massage her abdomen with the same and put a heat pack on it. I then suggested she take sesame seeds, morning and night if necessary (see details of remedies in the remedy section).

The following morning I had an email from her which consisted of about six lines of thank you thank you thank you thank you.

I am also asking you to ensure that you are drinking plenty of good quality water every day to clean out your kidneys too.

FOODS TO AVOID

There are some food groups best avoided in respect of 'prevention' and in particular for those not in good health, or with chronic diseases and allergies.

WHEAT & DAIRY

Wheat and dairy are 'inflammatory foods'. Inflammation in the body can affect arteries, joints, digestive and respiratory systems, bowels etc. Avoid highly processed carbohydrates such as sugar and flour as well as the thousands of products made from them, and also excess consumption of vegetable oils. These are perhaps the main contributors to inflammation in our body.

Dr Dwight Lundell, a cardiologist and heart surgeon of 25 years, said he did open heart surgery on some 5000 patients in that time and they all had one common denominator 'inflammation of the arteries'. His book *The Great Cholesterol Lie* is worth a read. He says if it were not for inflamed arteries cholesterol would flow freely. However, we all know that we must not consume foods which are going to contribute to 'bad cholesterol' either.

Unfortunately, only symptoms are treated in these conditions, and with drugs rather than treat the cause which is usually inflammation. Inflammation can be treated with diet. This is exactly what former US president Bill Clinton did. After heart surgery and further complications, he became aware of the effects of diet. You can hear interviews with him on YouTube where he speaks about his change in diet. You will hear it firsthand and you will also hear his doctor stating that heart disease is totally avoidable!

As I said before, 100 per cent PLANT based diets are not unusual to promote healing the body and getting the immune system working properly. There is no doubt whatsoever that when individuals start to increase their fresh food, especially with regular juicing of vegetables, green leaves and some fruits, it is very beneficial to health. Perhaps with the decline in soil quality and agricultural methods today, one cannot eat enough nutrients to satisfy the body's needs and juicing does compensate somewhat.

WHEAT

Wheat most definitely is not the same wheat we ate 50 years or more ago. Wheat can be stored in silos for a year where the grain is sprayed with pesticides, fungicides, etc., before it even gets to the flour mills. Remember the longer a plant is cut off from its life source the more the nutrients diminish!

The second consideration is that wheat contains gluten and this in itself is very clogging. Many people are gluten intolerant which may well be a result of a diet high in processed carbs made from wheat, such as bread, pasta, cereals, cakes, biscuits etc. It has also been suggested the intolerance is due to all of the sprays and chemicals used in the preservation of wheat, rather than the wheat itself. Allergies can be tested by coming off all wheat products for a month then re-introduce and observe any changes in symptoms and health. I advise all my clients to reduce their consumption of wheat but if they have any chronic health issues or symptoms I ask them to remove it altogether. There is no doubt today that overconsumption of this product contributes to health problems, allergies and chronic disease. My diabetic clients have all, without exception, benefited from more stable blood sugar readings after removing this completely from their diet, along with other dietary adjustments.

DAIRY/MEAT/CHICKEN

The way animals are farmed today, particularly beef and chicken, is not good for our health. These animals are given many drugs and hormone enhancers (often anabolic steroids), antibiotics and foods to 'fatten' them quickly. As a result the meat is high in fat and water, regardless of how lean the meat looks. Unless we buy hormone free, free range or organic chicken or grass fed meat from cows, we are eating meat from a very stressed animal probably full of various drugs/medications. These foods are also very inflammatory to the body and are best avoided as far as ill health and chronic disease is concerned. If we do eat meat/chicken and dairy products, ensure they are organic where the animals roam free and eat what nature intends them to eat.

Meat from animals which are 'free', like lamb and wild meats, I consider to be far safer than farmed animal meat!

FISH

Because of polluted waters, fish isn't as healthy as it used to be. Be particularly careful of large fish such as tuna as they are likely to be very high in mercury. The smaller fish are safer as far as pollution is concerned. Avoid farmed fish and eat local fresh where possible.

SUGARS

Sugars and fats are largely spoken of in relation to obesity but they can do far more harm than just contribute to weight gain. In simple terms sugar is acid; viruses, infections, cancers all love an acid environment and thrive in it. I repeat what I said earlier in quoting Dr Otto Warburg "disease cannot survive in an alkaline environment". Therefore, for prevention of health problems and to promote wellbeing, AVOID SUGAR. Natural sugars are better, but in moderation. At home we use raw honey, maple syrup and molasses.

ARTIFICIAL SWEETENERS

These cannot go unmentioned. The side effects and repercussions of their use are huge. Some have been withdrawn from the market eventually but others still lurk. I am asking you avoid these completely if you value your health. The side effects of aspartame can mimic symptoms such as those of multiple sclerosis and intake of it can seriously damage your health.

Aspartame is the common denominator for over 92 different health symptoms at the root of modern disease. The Aspartame Detoxification Program demonstrates the most effective way to reverse disease symptoms is removing the underlying cause – aspartame.

May I suggest you look at www.sweetpoison.com

GUIDANCE TO SOME ALTERNATIVE PRODUCTS

MOLASSES

We have all heard about the healing benefits of honey and the medicinal uses, so I am not going tell you what you may already know, but MOLASSES deserves a special mention because of its natural high mineral content. Take a look at these statistics.

Serving size 100 grams 290 calories		
Minerals		% daily value.
Calcium	205 mg	20%
Iron	4.72 mg	26%
Magnesium	242 mg	60%
Phosphorus	31 mg	3%
Potassium	1464 mg	61%
Sodium	37 mg	1%
Zinc	0.29 mg	1%
Copper	0.487 mg	24%
Manganese	1.53 mg	76%
Selenium	17.8 mcg	25%

It also contains some vitamins too		
Thiamin	0.041 mg	2%
Riboflavin	0.002 mg	0%
Niacin	0.93 mg	4%
Vitamin B6	0.67 mg	33%
Vitamin B12	0 mcg	0%
Folate	0 mcg	0%
Food Folate	0 5.6 mcg	~
Folic Acid	0 mcg	~
Dietary Folate Equivalents	0 mcg	~
Pantothenic Acid	0.804 mcg	8%

Our whole family takes molasses daily in one form or another and have done so for the past 25 years, a lot of my iron has come from this. This is also the product which I introduced to the lady with very low iron who was on medication! I don't suggest anyone takes themselves off any medication without the knowledge of their doctor and under supervision, but unless there is some reason why you should not introduce this to your diet, I highly recommend it – after all it is given to horses to make them strong!

NB: Don't cook molasses, like anything else, heat diminishes the nutrients. I stir a level teaspoon in soups and casseroles after taking from the heat and before serving. We also make a drink of one level teaspoon with hot water; milk can be added if desired. Or you can take it neat off the spoon, 1tsp three times a day if you suffer from tiredness, chronic fatigue and low energy.

FATS

In our home we use olive oil, ghee and butter. Olive oil however has a low tolerance of heat, therefore if you use it to cook, add a little butter or ghee which will help it heat a little better without becoming harmful. Frying and cooking in oil, is not the best way of cooking food apart from perhaps a stir fry using the minimum of oil.

Olive oil is best used as a dressing with lemon juice or by itself, as is flaxseed oil. We pour a good quality olive oil over our salads and vegetables.

Publicity over the decades has promoted other fats deemed as healthy but which have in many ways contributed to obesity and heart problems.

Indeed it is lack of good fats which has also been detrimental to health. Good fats are necessary for many bodily functions and in particular the brain. Take a look at Dr Terry Wahl who cured herself of advanced multiple sclerosis with diet and listen to what she has to say about healthy oils, especially omega 3. You will find her on YouTube. We need quite a lot of good fats in our diet. Good fats in food such as avocado, fish, nuts, omega 3/6 in the correct ratio, flaxseeds/oil and olive oil.

Often in my classes and workshops and individual consultations I am asked; if I can't buy all of these things which may be harmful to health, what do I buy instead? In organic shops there are many options but please note organic does not necessarily mean free from all additives. For example, a tin of organic kidney beans means the beans have been grown organically, it does not mean the liquid it is put into in the tin is organic, it may well be there is preservative or added salt in it. Likewise in organic wine, often sulphur dioxide is added which is a harmful additive and an asthma trigger. So please read your labels even as far as 'organic' is concerned.

Also please remember these are not living foods so keep them to a minimum.

Instead of	Alternatives
Wheat products – There are gluten free products in shops! I use buckwheat flour, sorghum flour and almond meal. There are many recipes available on the internet for all of these 'alternatives'.	
Bread	Try other grains such as buckwheat, sorghum, oat, or reduced wheat as in rye/organic and spelt.
Pasta.	Gluten free pasta such as organic buckwheat
Cereals	Raw organic oats, wheat-free muesli, quinoa flakes to make porridge, brown rice flakes.
Cakes & biscuits	Make your own with buckwheat or sorghum flour or oats, or almond meal and reduced sugar, although there are some gluten free ones on the market. Best to read and understand label ingredients, gluten free doesn't necessarily mean healthy but can in fact contain lots of additives.
White sugar	Raw sugar, rapadura sugar, raw honey.
Dairy products	
Milk	Almond milk, other nut milks, if you must buy diary try to buy organic un-homogenised.
Yogurt	Sheeps' yogurt is very nice.
Cheeses	Goats' cheese such as feta and chevre are nice or try making nut paste – it's easy.

Meat & Chicken	Very important to buy organic, free range, hormone free.
Home-made simple sauces instead of processed	
Cream sauce	Use 2tsps organic soured cream or crème fraiche diluted with natural stock and use as a cream sauce, such as for chicken. Onions and mushrooms can be added.
Tomato sauce	Make your own with a few ripe chopped tomatoes and either an small onion or garlic and simmer in a little hot water for a few minutes and mash or blend ... add herbs! Red capsicum can be added too.
Oils	Ghee, macadamia oil for cooking. Olive oil and flaxseed for dressings.

WHY ORGANIC FOOD

I prefer to call it 'natural food', food provided by nature untampered with by man! So instead of listening to all the pros and cons of whether organic is better or just a marketing ploy, consider this comparison:

Natural food provided by Mother Nature –v– man-made with chemicals!

Comparisons of nutrients emphasise the benefit of buying fresh local organic

ORGANIC VS CONVENTIONAL

Vegetables Type of Soil Mangement	Minerals (in milliequivalents)						
	Calcium	Magnesium	Potassium	Sodium	Manganese	Iron	Copper
Snap Beans							
Organic	40.5	60.0	99.7	8.6	60.0	227.0	69.0
Conventional	15.5	14.8	29.1	0.0	2.0	10.0	3.0
Cabbage							
Organic	60.0	43.6	148.3	20.4	13.0	94.0	48.0
Conventional	17.5	15.6	53.7	0.8	2.0	20.0	0.4
Lettuce							
Organic	71.0	49.3	176.5	12.2	169.0	516.0	60.0
Conventional	16.0	13.1	53.7	0.0	1.0	1.0	3.0
Tomatoes							
Organic	23.0	59.2	148.3	6.5	68.0	1938.0	53.0
Conventional	4.5	4.5	58.6	0.0	1.0	1.0	0.0
Spinach							
Organic	96.0	293.9	257.0	69.5	117.0	1584.0	0.0
Conventional	47.5	46.9	84.0	0.8	1.0	19.0	0.5
Research conducted by Firman E.Bear at Rutgers University in the Natural Gardner's Catalog (1995)							

I consider organic food to be the 'safest you can buy'. Even though it may not be totally 'chemical free' it is certainly a better option to food laced with a multitude of harmful chemicals.

PESTICIDES, FUNGICIDES & FERTILISERS

It has recently been stated that current regulations are inadequate to safeguard unborn children and children from potentially hazardous chemicals found in the environment and everyday items such as clothing, furniture and toys.

Apparently in the past seven years, the number of recognised chemical causes of neurodevelopmental disorders doubled. These include lead, arsenic, pesticides, such as DDT, solvents, methylmercury. These can be found in some fish and flame retardants that are often added to plastics and textiles, and manganese that can get into drinking water.

According to the Environmental Protection Agency 60 per cent of herbicides, 90 per cent of fungicides and 30 per cent of insecticides are known to **cause cancer.** Numerous studies suggest pesticides can contribute to infertility, birth defects, miscarriages and stillbirths, learning disorders, aggressive behaviour, cancer of the breast, prostate and lymphatic system.

I am sorry to say that we cannot rely on any authority to ensure the safety of our food because it is now impossible to test on thousands of chemicals used in food production and, even worse, the lethal cocktail of mixing chemicals which we ingest.

I am sure you are getting the picture by now; our food is grown in soil laced with chemicals and depleted of nutrients, it is then processed, preserved, coloured and laced with further chemicals, devoid of most if not all nutrients.

Dead food = ill health!

CHRONIC DISEASE, POOR HEALTH & DIET

When a client comes to see me with health problems I ask them to give me a list of everything they consume, from getting up in the morning to going to bed at night. What is their typical daily diet? At a glance I can usually see the foods they should not be eating, the lack of nutritious food, whether or not they are having enough of the right kind of fluids and whether or not their diet is out of balance.

WRONG DIET

What is an example of a diet typical of someone with chronic disease? This is not a judgement as most of the Western world has gone this way because we have all been misinformed.

Breakfast

A tea or coffee in the morning; followed by toast, cereal, both or nothing.

Mid-morning snack

Another tea or coffee and a biscuit/cake or perhaps nothing at all.

Lunch

A sandwich, sometimes with a processed meat like ham, maybe with salad.

Afternoon snack

Maybe another cup of tea and cake.

Dinner

Pasta, pizza, or sometimes meat or fish with vegetables.

So what is wrong with this?

What I look for when doing a nutritional assessment:

1. Inflammatory foods (chronic disease is inflammation in the body one way or another).
2. Acidic food & drink.
3. How much nutritious and living food they eat, which often isn't much.

Breakfast

Cereal & toast – (most likely includes wheat) – **inflammatory**.

Milk, probably in tea/coffee and on cereal – **inflammatory & acidic**.

Mid-morning snack

Biscuit/cake/pastry –(wheat, sugar, fats) – **inflammatory and acidic.**

Tea/coffee/milk – **acidic.**

Lunch

Sandwich/processed meat/cheese – (wheat, fats) – **inflammatory & acidic**.

Salad – **living food!**

Afternoon snack

Tea/biscuit –(wheat, sugars, fats) – **inflammatory & acidic**.

Dinner

Pasta, pizza –(wheat & fats) – **inflammatory and acidic**.

Meat/fish –(good protein, if it is from healthy source).

Vegetables – **living food**!

Do you see the picture?

And it is no surprise to me then when I test the acid/alkaline balance people with health problems are usually quite acidic. Most of the day people are consuming, at every meal, foods which can contribute to chronic disease. Food which causes inflammation in the body, and which puts a strain on our immune system. Food which is not sending nutrients into our blood stream and into our whole body to feed, nourish and heal. You would be surprised at the number of people who go days, even weeks without consuming any living food whatsoever. When I circle their list with all of the wrong foods and tick the correct foods, they too get the picture.

I ask clients, where is the protein we need to repair and renew our body. Where is the living food which gives us the vitamins, minerals and enzymes which we need to live a healthy life? Where are the fluids? A lot of people drink very little or no water.

STEPPING FORWARD TO A HEALTHY LIFE

If you want to step forward to a healthier life follow these steps.

If you care to make yourself a list of what your 'typical day's diet' comprises of, then make the necessary circles and ticks, you will clearly see where you need to make changes.

(Look at my 'typical day's diet' earlier in the book as an example). But bear in mind mine is to stay healthy. Much more nutritional saturation is required to speed up results in the case of chronic disease. Also bear in mind not all foods, even fresh, agree with everyone.

My initial suggestions for someone with chronic disease or long standing health problems would be:

Have a glass of water with fresh lemon juice on rising. All wheat would need to be removed from their diet.

Breakfast: I would introduce fresh fruit and eggs for breakfast (with healthy trimmings like spinach, tomato and avocado), or omelettes i.e. proteins and living food.

Mid-morning snack: A banana, apple or organic nuts and/or a homemade juice or smoothie (more living/nutritious food).

Lunch: Perhaps a salad with boiled eggs, or goats' cheese, or wild salmon (protein and living food).

Afternoon snack: A piece of fruit, herb tea or fresh juice (living food).

Dinner: A good quality piece of fish or chicken, lentils or chickpeas, (initially avoiding red meat), with lots of vegetables, especially leafy greens (protein and living food).

Just be careful not to overdo the protein. Younger people, who still have a lot of growing to do, usually need more protein than adults. Around 0.8gm per 1kg of body weight is a good guide per day.

In this example we have removed all sugars, wheat and most dairy and introduced nutritious/living food every time a person puts something in their mouth. How easy is this?

For people who are at work I encourage them at weekends to buy lots of fresh fruit, salads and vegetables at the local market (organic or spray free if possible). Salads can be washed and stored in the fridge, including tomatoes; beetroot boiled or grated, also carrot. How easy is it in the morning to put these together in a sealed bowl to take with you? A couple of eggs can be boiling while you are doing this to take with you for lunch. Include an apple or banana, a dish of nuts and dried sulphur-free fruit and you have lots of good food to take with you. I also encourage clients to make a large juice or protein drink and put it in a thermos flask and take that with them too.

The extra emphasis with chronically sick patients is to do lots of juicing throughout the day. It doesn't mean you have to stand several times a day making them. I have some large glass bottles with caps and every morning, whilst I am chopping and slicing our fruit salad for breakfast I also do my fruit and greens for the juices. I make about a litre and half of green juice with pineapple, apple, banana and lots of green leaves and herbs, and the same amount of a protein drink with raw egg yolk, a dash of honey, mixed berries, banana and a handful of whole raw almonds and sometimes add a protein powder like pea protein as well. These I bottle, pop in the fridge and we drink throughout the day between our meals.

I can say with confidence that in every case, a client with chronic disease has achieved very good results within the month. Diabetics have stabilised blood sugars (even if it has taken a while later for their doctor to have the confidence to remove medication), cholesterol levels have lowered quite rapidly, weight loss has been attained without trying, joint pain and migraines have disappeared, energy levels have increased and quality of life has started to return.

In respect of children's health, there are usually, within days, noticeable signs of changes in things such as behaviour, concentration, reduction and even elimination of asthma attacks, and as their immune system builds up, less infections, coughs and colds etc.

With chronic disease it is good to do intense nutrition as mentioned, eliminating inflammatory foods – all wheat and preferably all animal foods – at the same time having lots of living foods each meal and lots and lots of daily juicing. This approach will really give the body a kick start and trigger the healing processes. Time and time again my clients come and tell me 'my specialist says', or 'my doctor says' "keep doing what you are doing it's working", and in the case of a special cancer client "keep doing what you are doing, your immune system is working again".

Other foods can be introduced eventually, but certainly not processed foods. Re-introducing a good quality ancient grain bread or 'oat' bread with basic ingredients, oats, oat bran, olive oil, water and maybe a little salt is not going to hurt. Neither will some home-made, wheat-free fruit and nut bars, or home-made biscuits with good ingredients for an occasional treat but occasional is the key. Even occasional gluten-free, wheat-free pasta isn't going to kill you but the main source of our daily diet needs to be good wholefoods ensuring we have lots of living foods too.

In the case of keeping healthy and preventing disease I take the same approach, but also suggest the alternatives mentioned in Step 2 'Guidance of some alternatives'. Reasonably healthy people who are just wanting to improve their health and avoid chronic disease and ill health in later life can cope with eating a more 'normal diet' as long as they remove processed foods and decrease or remove the inflammatory foods mentioned earlier, and of course, increase their nutrition. My typical daily diet is an example. We occasionally have a little oat bread, eat some organic meat/chicken although not a lot, but I do make home-made healthy chocolate treats and desserts so you do not have to deprive yourself completely. Even those on a strict diet because of chronic disease can eat some healthy treats daily – in fact it is these little treats that help people adjust. (I will give a few examples at the end of the book).

It is easy to look at your current meals, see where the changes need to be made and do it. If you cannot cope with making the full change start with breakfast for a week, then work on the snacks or lunch. The important thing is DO IT!

SUPPLEMENTS AND SUPERFOODS

The simplicity of it is moving to a wholesome fresh diet with variations of all the wonderful living foods available to us which will feed and nourish our body properly. You can use 'superfoods' if you wish, or introduce them later but I do not want to mention them at this stage because there are those who think if they take lots of vitamins and minerals and other supplements and superfoods, this will save them the trouble of eating good healthy meals all of the time. But it is also very expensive. Let's get into a new habit of buying and eating good food, and include some of these if you wish but not instead of!

There are some who prefer the support of supplements, whilst they adjust their diet. The most important thing is to focus on the food and healthy changes as soon as possible. I am quite aware that we can become very depleted in some vitamins and minerals depending on our health problem, our kind of diet, soil etc. The basic supplementation I would take into consideration is zinc, omega 3, a good probiotic, vitamin D, depending on the condition, and in some circumstances a good multi mineral/vitamin for a while.

ZINC

I must make a special mention of zinc. My good friend and mentor told me many years ago to take zinc occasionally (to top up) as zinc is in very few foods. We lose more than we can eat, especially if we are very active because we lose a lot of zinc through perspiration. I have always remembered that and eventually I did quite a lot of study into the mineral zinc. What stuck in my mind was its involvement in so many bodily functions. I also read that women depleted in zinc can have difficulty in conceiving, and also that it is important in the development of the brain of the foetus and can affect learning abilities too.

Many years later I was helping a lady who could not conceive and I was reminded by a medical colleague that sometimes all that is needed is a boost of zinc. I shared this with the lady (who by the way was on a good diet) and by coincidence or not she conceived within a few months and now has a beautiful baby.

I was also reminded of the effects of zinc and the brain and recently read a research paper on ADHD which also indicated that a lot of children with these symptoms are found to be low in zinc, and supplementation along with minerals has sometimes made a difference.

So there are instances when our body does need that extra help over and above diet, but I believe short term not long. We have to remember; supplements do come out of processing factories in the main and can have additives, coatings, preservatives etc., so it is important to read ingredient labels on these too.

But rather – Let Food be your medicine!

SUMMARY OF STEP 2

- Buy the best quality local fresh produce, preferably organic
- Consider eating some 'raw meals'
- Introduce juicing for added nutrition
- Include some super foods in your diet/juices
- Try nut milks and cheeses
- Try to eat 80/20 alkaline food to acid
- Try to avoid wheat products
- Try to reduce diary but buy organic or try goats' and sheeps' produce
- Buy organic meats and chicken
- Avoid large fish to avoid mercury
- Cut out sugars
- Change to healthy fats

CHAPTER 4

STEP 3
CHILDREN

I have decided to do a separate section for children as I am constantly told my child won't eat what I give it, or my child won't eat, or my child only wants to eat bread or cake and won't eat fruit and vegetables etc. When I see what some people put into their supermarket trolleys, all the different coloured bottles of drinks or cola, packets of snacks, crisps, biscuits, cereals, tins of food, little or no fresh fruit and vegetables, I cringe. If only people understood what they are buying and what these foods do to your health.

The symptoms these children will experience apart from hyperactivity and concentration problems will probably be headaches, tummy aches, constipation, lots of colds and sore throats or even more severe symptoms and allergic reactions like asthma and eczema, their immune systems will be weakened and ultimately will lead to ill health, obesity, diabetes and other chronic diseases. Children are now suffering from arthritis at an early age and apparently cancer is now one of the biggest killers of children in Australia.

Some mums will go part way to improve diets for their family but they tell me they still buy such and such because their children like it or because they won't eat anything else. Well, I have some good news for all of you mums; you can change a child's appetite in less than two weeks!

Which is better?

Giving your child sugar (processed chocolates, sweets, biscuits, cakes, snacks etc. etc.) because your child likes it and because you feel awful depriving your child of these 'treats';

OR

Refusing to buy these foods, and thereby protecting your child from harm. Instead you will give them long-term good health and maybe even save their life.

I will quote a heading from an article I was reading on cancer – it said

'Loving your child to death with sugar'

The choice is yours!

A few years ago I watched a documentary on TV which was a televised experiment. A family of five (mum, dad and three school age children) volunteered to eat no processed foods for six weeks. The whole family were overweight and probably heading for serious health problems if they continued as they were. They all had medical checks and blood tests before and after the experiment.

At the beginning of the experiment the mother emptied her home of all processed foods before the children got in from school. There was just a bowl of fruit placed on the table. When the children arrived home the three of them went straight to the fridge and cupboards looking for their usual snacks and drinks and in a very demanding agitated tone asked where everything was. The mum showed them the fruit bowl and told them that was all they were allowed before dinner. The children became very abusive and of course it distressed the mother and she felt awful. This persisted each day including complaining about their 'new' meals free of junk. On around the third day they came home and went straight to the fruit bowl, helped themselves to a piece of fruit and quietly went away and ate it. Within a few days they accepted without argument their new way of life and diet!

At the end of the six weeks, apart from enjoying their good food, they had all lost weight, had more energy, were a lot calmer, a lot nicer to each other, slept better and all of their blood tests showed a dramatic improvement.

I read of a similar experiment done in a young offenders' institution where every offender on the programme not only changed personality, but became very remorseful about their crimes and couldn't believe they had committed them.

I would also like to mention an experiment which was conducted in England some years ago, which was again televised, and a few years later, I also saw it on Australian TV.

Parents and teachers of a class of school children (I think they were about six years old) agreed to take part in a one-week experiment. Again it was not to feed the children with any processed food/additives whatsoever.

Parents and teachers reported their disbelief at the changes in these children, they reported they were calmer, much better behaved, slept better and there was a huge increase in test results in school.

On the last day of the experiment it showed the children sitting during the morning listening to their teacher read a story, without any disturbance whatsoever. At lunchtime they held a children's party for them which included all the typical party food of cakes, biscuits, savouries, different coloured icings and decorations etc. Within thirty minutes of eating the party food the children were totally uncontrollable. They were noisy, badly behaved, would not sit down even for a story. The teachers could not do anything but watch in disbelieve. Thirty minutes is all it took to affect each child's behaviour.

What more can I say!

So parents, have you heard of the saying you have to be cruel to be kind?

For your child's sake, for their future health, wellbeing and longevity, you have to put up with the aggravation for a short while for a lifetime's benefit! But will you do it?

Following steps 1 and 2 is where you begin to make those very important changes.

SOME TIPS –

- Young children do not like to be faced with large meals, better to let them have second helpings if needed than pile too much on the plate to start with. This is also a good tip for adults too. If they are old enough, better still to let them serve themselves.

If I offered my child say an apple or banana they would probably refuse it, but if I chopped different fruits, different colours and maybe even different shapes and put them on a platter they would run to choose their own selection. I do the same with my grandchildren, I show them the platter as I walk to the table, their little faces light up and they run to me to get some.

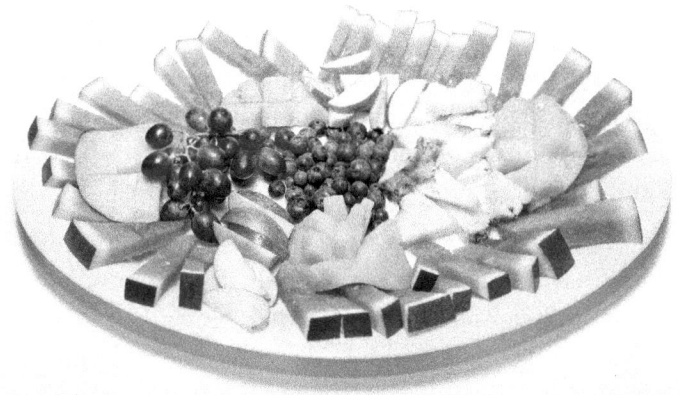

- When I make a snack or a light lunch for them, as I did sometimes with my own children, I do the same thing. I get a large platter and decorate it with small pieces of different foods for example;

Carrot, celery, grapes, mango, watermelon, avocado, apple and perhaps additive free crackers with cheese or nut paste on them. Children can't wait to pick up to try the small pieces and the different colours. Sometimes to make it more substantial I will make small triangular sandwiches from oat bread with cheese, or avocado and tomato, or egg.

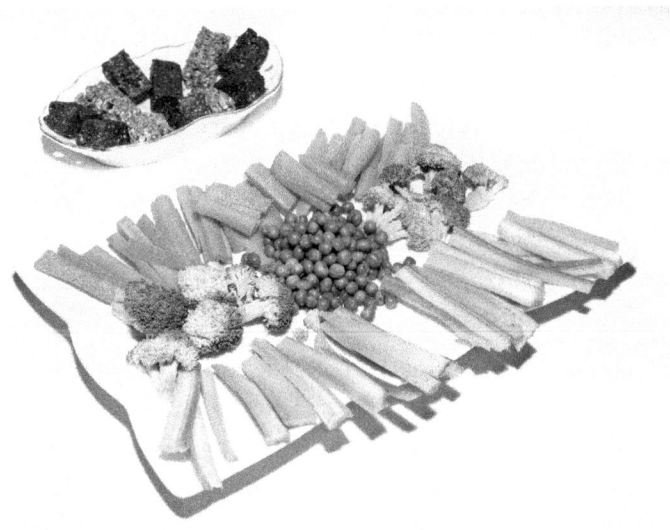

- For dinner you can do the same with different coloured steamed vegetables like carrots, peas, broccoli, sweet corn, sweet potato and then a little protein like organic chicken strips or a lamb cutlet. Small healthy chocolate treats can be served after lunch and dinner or as snacks.

It is also very important to follow appetites, but of course not to confuse with cravings for sugar, chocolate, and addictive fast foods. If we have an appetite for something it usually means our body needs it, i.e. the minerals, vitamins and enzymes.

I remember years ago when I was first introduced to homemade carrot juice, I could have drank buckets full of it. Possibly my body was lacking vitamin A or beta-carotene or some other mineral or vitamin in carrots. When I'd had enough and could go days without it, I knew my body had got what it needed. We all should listen to our body in that way and should not force children to eat something they do not want. Bear in mind they may not want it because we haven't made it look appetising, or it is too much for them, or indeed they just do not want it at that moment in time.

I was at a retreat recently where we were reminded every morning to ask ourselves 'what does my body feel like doing today', it may be a gentle walk, it may be we are bursting with energy and feel like a good work out in a gym. How harmful it would be if we felt tired and our body needed to rest and we ignored the feeling and went and ran a marathon! We must listen to our body as well as our appetite. When you are preparing food for the family it is good to ask what they would like to eat for such and such a meal – obviously you don't want to prepare different meals for everyone but you may be able to incorporate something to please them all.

So with young children, if you are preparing food to make it look appetising and appealing, do not worry if they only want to eat carrot or celery for a few days, as long as it is not a processed harmful food, that's okay, they probably need it and you will soon know when they have had enough. The exception to this of course is if your child is unwell, needs a medical check, or is not just attention seeking, which needs to be dealt with differently.

I do not have a sweet tooth at all, I hardly ever eat desserts. However, if suddenly I felt like something sweet, I would have a little as my body probably needs a little natural sugar or something to boost my serotonin levels or similar. As long as I have a little of something natural, it will not create a craving for me and will satisfy. Alternatively, if someone has an appetite for sweet things, sometimes giving a little protein will suppress it. There are some very easy healthy recipes for snacks and nibbles – and for those with a sweet tooth – which you can make at home. You can even buy or make healthy ice-cream and yogurts without additives and all good fats!

SUMMARY OF STEP 3

- Keep away from additives and processed food
- Be firm
- Introduce fruit and healthy snacks
- For children, make portions/pieces small, colourful and attractive so you don't over face them
- Listen to appetites
- Don't force eating with bribes or threats

Introduction to steps 4 and 5

These next steps are very important for our protection too. Often we shrug our shoulders at what happens in the environment and what is put into products we use for our home and personal use, but our health is very much affected by these chemicals and there is much we can do about it, particularly for ourselves, which cumulatively can also help the environment.

CHAPTER 5

STEP 4
HOW CHEMICALS IN OUR TOILETRIES AND COSMETICS AFFECT OUR HEALTH

I read an article that suggested we ladies use some 500 chemicals on our skin every day between showering, hair washing, moisturising, perfumes and make-up, toothpaste, oral care, deodorants, sprays etc.

The main thing to consider is that our skin is part of our excretory system, not only does it pass out toxins from our body through perspiration, but it can also absorb whatever touches our skin and which goes straight into our bloodstream and all around our body into each organ!

I was first alerted to these dangers whilst holiday in the Canary Islands some 20 years ago. One day I picked up the local freebie newspaper called the Canarian weekly, flicking through it my attention was drawn to an article which was in the 'Health' section, headed 'The Danger Zone' and in large capital letters the subject heading was 'Making an informed choice about your personal care and health'. The first paragraph read:

'Harmful by inhalation. Harmful if swallowed, Irritating to eyes.

Irritating to respiratory system. Irritating to skin. Corrosive to hair and hair follicles. May cause sensitisation by inhalation. Accumulative to organs. In case of contact with eyes or skin rinse immediately with plenty of water and seek medical advice. **Wear protective clothing and safety glasses.**' (I still have a copy of the article in my file!)

I couldn't wait to see what they were referring to but then I was dumfounded when I read on –

Who would think that all the above warnings would have anything to do with ingredients commonly found in almost every personal care product in your home – shampoo, shower gel, conditioner, toothpaste, baby bath, baby lotion (yes it is also in children's personal care products), shaving cream, bubble bath etc.

The additive(s) was sodium lauryl sulphate (SLS) and sodium laureth sulphate (SLES) – and also carries this warning: 'SLS & SLES are known carcinogens (they cause cancer) and other health problems attributed to it also include dermatitis, eczema, psoriasis, retarded healing and they are now known to cause cataracts in adults and impede eye development in children.

Repeated exposure can cause major dysfunction in the brain, heart, lungs and liver via constant absorption through the skin.

Where is the logic in putting these harmful chemicals in skin products when they causes skin problems? Why are these chemicals known to corrode hair and hair follicles in shampoos? By the way it is so strong it is used to degrease car engines and scrub garage floors! Apparently SLS and SLES can stay in the body for up to five days. It easily penetrates the skin and can affect heart, liver lungs and brain. You know there are thousands of chemicals in personal care products and only a fraction, if any, are tested properly for safety.

Needless to say after reading this article I was determined to eliminate chemicals for our personal use and in our home. It was difficult 20 years ago because alternatives were few and far between. In fact I could only find one shampoo from America that didn't contain any nasties. Today however, there are many brands of personal care products, both commercially produced and home–made products sold locally. I am trying different ones all the time. There is none in particular which I would recommend except to buy natural to protect yourself and your family.

Let's take a look at a few more chemicals so that you are clear about the harm they cause to our health and you can understand clearly what you need to avoid when you are shopping.

INGREDIENT	SIDE EFFECTS	USES
Butylene glycol *	Ingestion may cause renal damage vomiting, drowsiness, depression coma and death	Hairspray, setting lotions, Cosmetics
1,4-Dioxane preparations	Hormone disruption, mimics oestrogen, kidney, liver, neuro and Cardiovascular toxicity. Lowered sperm Counts, stress related illness, teratogenic; Carcinogenic	Pesticides, detergent
Formaldehyde	Eye, nose and throat irritation, coughing Nose bleeds, affects liver, respiratory and Immune systems, causes skin problems	Mascara, nail polish, soap, hair restorer
	Reproductive system and is neurotoxic, It can also cause asthma and It is on the NIH hazards list and is teratogenic, carcinogenic	Anti-aging creams shampoo, bubble baths and deodorants
Parabens	Can mimic the action of the female hormone Oestrogen which can encourage breast tumours	Deodorant and cosmetics
Phthalates	Linked to birth defects and reproduction	Plasticizing ingredients in many products
Musks	Skin irritation, hormone disruption, cancer	Used in fragrances
Artificial fragrances	One of the top 5 allergens causing asthma	
Toluene	Anaemia, lowered blood cell count, liver kidney damage, may affect foetus.	Made from petroleum Found in many fragrances
Mineral oil, paraffin	These products coat your clogging pores and create a build-up of toxins. Slow cellular development which can cause earlier signs of aging and are suspected to cause cancer and disruption to hormonal activity.	

Amongst known carcinogens are ethylene oxide, dioxane, nitrosamines, formaldehyde, and acrylamide!

In England a few years ago I was asked by a neighbour if I could help a friend's four-year-old child. This child was being taken to hospital daily to have fresh dressings put on her bleeding eczema. This had been going on for about three weeks. I never met the parent or the child but I did put written 'advice' together for the mother which included guidance on chemical-free toiletries, household and laundry products so that the child's clothes, towels and bedclothes were free of chemicals on her skin, as well as giving the mother guidance on the specific eczema-causing additives in food and drink. It was simple, easy to follow, one page 'advice'. The feedback from the neighbour was that it had made a big difference.

I do not normally like to work this way, if you like it was a quick first aid help. I would have much preferred to sit down with the mum and give her the full picture of how much she could help her child.

Remember the skin is part of our elimination system. It is often no good putting creams and treatments on skin problems if the underlying cause is toxicity in the body which is trying to get out. We have to deal with what's going on in the inside!

Other cases have resulted in people feeling very itchy all over, and after eliminating allergic reactions to food, it was established that they used shower gels which cause a lot of skin problems (all of which contain the SLS and SLES mentioned previously).

When we were children we used soap; soap for washing, soap for hair washing, we had no deodorants or body moisturisers, no harmful sunscreens. If you look at the shelves upon shelves of toiletries and cosmetics lining chemists and supermarket shelves, they are in their hundreds, and the chemicals are in their thousands.

SUNSCREENS

As a teenager and young woman spreading her wings, I couldn't wait to get to the Mediterranean for some sun as we saw so little of it in England, and yes I did use oils and sunscreen, because I trusted they protected me. Now we know better, we don't use any or just a natural one. Obviously, we all take precautions to cover and not to burn but not to deprive ourselves of the all-important vitamin D from the sun which is our best source.

Isn't it crazy all of these years we have been told to wrap up and slap up (as they say in Australia), both of which have resulted in deprivation of the sun and subsequently vitamin D deficiencies, and putting endless chemicals on our skin both of which are likely to have contributed in the massive increase in cases of skin cancer. There is a lot of information and evidence available for those wanting to look into this further.

DEODORANTS & ANTI-PERSPERANTS

A special mention is needed regarding the use of deodorants and antiperspirants.

We have pores under our arm which not only allows the body to sweat to cool down but also to release toxins (the smell we get is bacteria). What do you think happens to those toxins if we block the pores with deodorants and antiperspirants? Where do the toxins go? If these products are made with chemicals, they seep through our pores into our body, our bloodstream, our lymphatic system!

Have you ever noticed small sore lumps under the arm occasionally? These are blocked lymphatics! The lymphatic system runs down the arms, under the arms, across the chest/breast and down to the liver. If the lymphatics are blocked in that area, the toxins can accumulate in the chest/breast area!

I have read recently that since the introduction of deodorants and particularly antiperspirants, there has been a rise in breast cancer in both men and women!

Ladies bras', especially boned, tight ones also restrict the lymphatics in the breast area. I recall Don Tolman saying if you don't want breast lumps of any kind, don't wear deodorant, don't wear a bra and go for a run! He said the men would be happy! Joking aside it makes sense, not only you don't restrict lymphatic drainage but by bouncing (whether on a mini-trampoline in your front room or a jog in the garden), the bouncing helps move any blockages in the lymphatics and we should do this daily! There is supportive underwear made today without restriction and bones and in natural fibres which is much more comfortable and healthier than most underwear.

All that is needed is to wash regularly in the under arm area to keep the pores open and wipe away any unpleasant aromas.

SPRAYS

Hair, deodorant, perfume, cologne (as well as all household sprays which will be mentioned later), these chemicals go into the atmosphere and the air we breathe; we inhale them. When we inhale them, as well as irritating our respiratory system and maybe contributing to such allergies as asthma, these chemicals pass from our lungs into our bloodstream and to every organ of our body!

Yes, I am repeating the process – no matter how we use chemicals in food or products, they end up in our body one way or another. It is really important to keep emphasising this so that everyone will realise just how much our body has to cope with so we understand the relationship of chemicals and poor health.

TOOTHPASTE

On fluoridated toothpaste there is a 'POISON' warning not to be swallowed. Adults may be able to adhere to this warning, but can children? My recollection is that they swallow a lot. At home we buy fluoride free toothpaste which is usually made from bi-carbonate of soda, herbs and peppermint. These can be found in supermarkets and can also be made at home easily and cheaply.

HAIR CARE

Many natural shampoos and conditioners and even hair colourings can now be found both in health stores and at some markets. I have used a 'herb' based colour/highlighter for over 20 years and everyone thinks my hair is a natural colour. Like all other products, read your labels. Suppliers are getting the message and state clearly on their packaging; 'free from chemicals, BPAs, parabens etc. etc.

SOAPS AND SHOWER GELS

There is much natural soap now readily available with different natural fragrances. A lot are made with an olive oil or macadamia nut base and some with goat's milk. We like olive oil based soaps and buy original Castile liquid soap which we use as our shower gel.

MOISTURISERS

Don Tolman says 'don't put on your skin what you wouldn't put in your mouth'. Well that makes sense doesn't it, because whatever we eat or use ends up in our blood stream affecting our whole body. There are some really lovely natural moisturisers available these days. Give your skin a good dry brush to remove dead skin, before getting into the shower. A good exfoliate if you need one is fine sea salt mixed into a paste with olive oil. After showering, rinsing and drying, apply a natural moisturiser. Your skin will love it, absorb it, and at first it will absorb a lot of it until your skin is no longer thirsty then you will use a reduced amount. Try it!

MAKE-UP

I am now able to find natural mineral powders, foundations, eye shadows, lipsticks and much more, even nail varnishes without the dreaded formaldehyde in them which is great news! If you don't have time to shop, go online, everything we need in a natural product is out there.

I have covered this section briefly to give you an insight as to the number of chemicals we may be using in one day. We may have used them for many years not realising the amounts or the risks we have been taking – and certainly not the health implications.

Can you now begin to see the many thousands of chemicals we have bombarded ourselves with both orally and externally over many years? Our immune systems have been on full alert for so long they have become so weakened they cannot function properly. You can change this with all the awareness you now have obtained.

Dr Samuel Epstein, who is a well-respected professional in cancer prevention, is an expert on toxins. In an interview with Dr Mercola he expressed several pressing health dangers, one of which was about nano-particles used in cosmetics. Some of these nano-particles he says are so dangerous they are becoming known as 'universal asbestos'. He said they are touted as reducing wrinkling and firming up the skin but 'pose an extraordinarily dangerous and unrecognised public health hazards'.

He said there is evidence of them penetrating the skin, invading underlying blood vessels, getting into the bloodstream and producing toxic effects. He said there is evidence of, degenerative disorders in the brain and nerve damage. He referred to these products as 'the most dangerous types of products in the whole cosmetic industry'.

According to Dr Epstein, in 2008 a British Royal Commission report warned that products that contain nanoparticles pose very, very high toxic risks.

SUMMARY STEP 4

- READ INGREDIENT LABELS ON ALL PRODUCTS
- USE NATURAL COSMETICS/TOILETRIES, MAKE-UP, HAIR PRODUCTS
- USE NATURAL SUNSCREENS
- AVOID SPRAYS OF ANY KIND
- DO NOT USE DEODORANTS AND ANTIPERSPIRANTS

CHAPTER 6

STEP 5
HOW CHEMICALS IN THE HOME AFFECT OUR HEALTH

This chapter is again designed to give you an awareness of the health dangers in the home. Much more in-depth detail is readily available to those who wish to know more.

Let me give you a scenario.

A child has eczema. The child is treated with perhaps a chemical pharmaceutical cream to try to sooth and heal the symptoms on the outside, which may be cracked, sore and bleeding.

My mentor said to me many years ago, what comes out of the skin is a sign of what's going on inside the body! Won't chemical creams absorb into the body, thus adding more toxins? It may be helpful in soothing, but it may be making the problem worse!

The child is bathed or showered in tap water (which may contain fluoride and other harmful substances), bath and shower-gel type products containing chemicals are used to wash the child! The child is dried on a towel washed in a chemical based laundry powder, and maybe even fabric conditioner containing the dreaded formaldehyde! The child will then be dressed in clothes washed in the same products and will then sleep on sheets and pillow cases washed in the same chemical based products.

This same child may be eating many hundreds of chemicals found in food and drink!

This child is possibly also exposed to many household products used in cleaning the home!

Do you see the full picture? How do we help this child? We reverse everything we have mentioned, removing every chemical orally, externally, inhaled, and give the child living food, ensuring she has the correct minerals and vitamins needed not only to heal the skin but to heal the body and prevent any such problems in the future.

A gentleman I knew had a constant rash and itching on his elbows – he did not know what caused it and could not find relief. It eventually came to light that the he used to lie on the carpet, propped up by his elbows, and the wife used to sprinkle a chemical deodorant on the floor because of doggy smells!

EXAMPLES OF HAZARDOUS HOUSEHOLD CHEMICALS

Ammonia	A volatile chemical that is damaging to eyes, respiratory tract and skin, commonly found in multipurpose cleaners and oven cleaners.
Chlorine bleaches	A strong corrosive that irritates or burns the skin, eyes and respiratory tract. Toxic to the brain and nervous system. Commonly found in toilet cleaners, bathroom mould removers, auto dishwasher powders and bleaches.
Petroleum based detergents	Causes irritation of the skin, lungs, sinuses and eyes. Commonly found in laundry powders and liquids, multipurpose cleaners, toilet and bathroom cleaners and pre-wash stain removers.
Synthetic fragrances	Mostly petroleum derived – found in all types of cleaners. Ethylene glycol, glycol ethers and glycol esters are synthetic solvents used in paints, lacquers, resins, printing inks, cleaning fluids and anti-freeze and additives in aviation fuel. This solvent group is highly toxic and women who use solvents have twice as many miscarriages as other women. They also rapidly diffuse through the skin and through ordinary rubber gloves while the aromatic solvents can cause brain damage at high doses and be addictive.

Phenol/Phenyl	Carbolic acid. Very toxic, kills beneficial bacteria in sewerage treatment works and repeated exposure can damage the brain, liver kidneys and spleen. Found in disinfectants.
Formaldehyde	Also known as formalin, it is the most common air pollutant in houses. It can cause eye, nose and throat irritations, coughing, asthmas, shortness of breath, nausea, vomiting, skin rashes, weakening of the immune system and headaches. Found in fabric softeners. A small amount of formaldehyde gas escapes from all formaldehyde products such as upholstery, foam insulation, laminated wood, particleboard furniture and permanent press fabrics.

Therefore, here are some alternatives.

Health stores now sell a good selection of natural household, laundry and cleaning products and even supermarkets are selling products with less harmful chemicals in some areas.

LAUNDRY

There are now a few more natural laundry products in supermarkets, health stores and some farmers' markets. Personally, I use a half mix of bi-carbonate of soda with the same amount of 'baking soda' which is 100% natural which I buy in the supermarket and I have either eucalyptus or lavender for fragrances and antiseptic.

CLEANING

We mainly use white vinegar in water, and again use lavender or eucalyptus for fragrances. We also use bi-carbonate of soda in water as a cleaner, or sometimes mix it with a natural soap like the castile soap or a natural dishwashing liquid and make a paste to clean sinks and baths. Lemon juice can be used as a bleach or disinfectant too.

Beeswax makes good furniture polish both for wood and leather, including handbags and shoes.

A good degreaser for the kitchen is one part white vinegar to two parts water plus a little liquid natural soap. Add baking soda to make a more abrasive cleaner.

For floor washing, a little vinegar in a bucket of water with a little lemon juice for fragrance makes a good cleaner.

MOULD

Vinegar can kill mould. It is very important to keep mould at bay – this can be highly toxic in the home and needs to be avoided. Particular attention should be made to pillows, mattresses and blankets, especially pillows as they can become very toxic from perspiration. Pillows which start to go discoloured should be thrown out immediately.

I recently read about a lady staying in a hotel who could not get to sleep. She could not settle at all. She opened windows, tossed and turned and no matter where she lay in the bed she could not sleep. She decided to check the pillows and removed the pillow cases to find they were very stained and she realised the toxic fumes she was inhaling when lying on these pillows was the problem.

New furniture, carpets and even newly decorated rooms can give off a lot of toxic fumes for some weeks, even months. Ensure such rooms are well ventilated.

ALUMINIUM COOKWARE

Another hazard in the home to be aware of is the use of plastics and aluminium, especially in connection with food preparation and storage. It has been widely known for some time to avoid using aluminium saucepans as aluminium is known to be neurotoxic. Therefore, I would suggest using glass/Pyrex type pans, ceramic or cast iron.

PLASTICS & FOOD STORAGE

- Male sperm counts worldwide have been reduced by 50 per cent in the past half century.
- Increasing abnormalities in embryos, genitals, more miscarriages.
- Increased number of men seeking breast reduction surgery.
- Girls entering puberty much younger!

Plastics, amongst other things, are a huge endocrine disruptor. Apart from causing damage to the environment, oceans, coral reefs, they are one of the worse contributors to toxicity in our body. NB: Remember that most of our toiletries and cosmetics also come in plastic containers too.

Avoid using cling wraps, aluminium foils, plastic containers for food and drink. Again it has been widely published that the BPA's in plastics are highly toxic. It is linked to hormone disruption, diabetes, breast cancer and much more. Tests around the globe on reducing fertility rates are connected to these chemicals. There are some BPA-free plastics available, as in baby formulae bottles, but glass is better. If you must use the wrappings, at least first wrap the food in baking paper so the plastic or foil does not touch the food. There is a good selection of glass storage containers and jars available and even if they have plastic lids, I cover with baking paper before placing the lid.

EMFs/RADIATION

Well over 20 years ago my dear friend and mentor said to me not to have a mobile phone, don't use cordless phones in the house, don't watch colour TV for more than 20 minutes at a time, and sit as far away as possible from TVs. Don't sit in front of a computer for long periods and don't use a microwave oven. She told me they were all dangerous to health, before anyone ever questioned the use of these products!

I did not use a mobile at the time, I ensured our home phones remained corded, i.e. not the ones you can walk around with like a mobile, we dumped our microwave oven and our TV was small screen and we limited use. Our business used computers and it was difficult then as is now to operate without them but we were able to buy protective screens at the time to limit radiation exposure to our staff and to ourselves.

At that time I did not have time to research the whys and wherefores, but my friend was always so accurate in her intuition that I followed and felt no need to check for myself. Her words have proven accurate once again.

MICROWAVE OVENS

These were banned in Russia in the 1976. In 1989 a Swiss food scientist made some worrying discoveries about microwave ovens. He was effectively gagged by the manufacturers who used trade laws to get the Swiss courts to muzzle him and he was prohibited from publicly declaring or writing that microwave ovens were dangerous to health. We are not going into details here; you can search "detrimental effects of microwave cooking" and see the evidence for yourself. A report published by 'What Doctors don't tell you.com website' in March 2000 is headed *Microwave Ovens – a recipe for cancer*. 'Ten-year-old evidence suppressed by the Swiss courts, shows that food from a microwave can cause worrying changes in your blood.' It includes warnings such as the effects on heating milk and infant formulae. Please seriously consider the implications of using these ovens. Everyone I have shared this information with has thrown out their microwave ovens after reading the evidence.

MOBILE TELEPHONES

Many years ago and not that long after my friend passed on these warnings, two of our neighbours got tumours, one in the head and the other in the ear/throat area. The first gentleman in his fifties told me it was the second time these tumour had developed; the first time was a few years previous. It was the side of his head where he used his mobile telephone, and he used it a lot. In those days the mobile was rather large and when the top part was held to the ear, the bottom part would curve round the throat towards the mouth, similar to that of a handset today.

The other gentleman was a young man in his thirties, the father of a new born baby. This young man I used to see regularly leaving his home, already on his mobile and often return home at night, still using his mobile. My thoughts then were 'why not make the call in your drive before you leave instead of driving with one hand' really thinking of the dangers of driving and talking on the phone. Little did I realise there was another danger lurking. I really don't know if this young man survived as we left the country around the same time.

In more recent years I watched a documentary on Australian TV, it was an interview with a neurosurgeon. The part I remember vividly was his comments about the dramatic increase in the number of operations on brain tumours in recent years. When he was asked what he thought the cause of the rise in brain tumours was he said he was in no doubt whatsoever it was mobile telephones. He stressed the importance of limiting use, keeping conversations short and using speaker phones. It would make sense to take such precautions.

I saw a head scan done in some research and when the person put the mobile telephone up to the ear the whole area around the ear glowed red which I understood to be brain cells being burned. I understand the penetration can be up to two inches (5cm).

I believe other symptoms related to the use of mobiles are ear problems, vision problems, headaches, dizziness and vertigo.

COMPUTERS

Seizures in children have been widely connected with overuse of computers, especially when games became the rage. Nowadays, computers are no longer just desktops linked to the telephone cable for internet, but wireless is now the way to go with more and more use of laptops and iPads.

It has recently been argued that the new 'wireless' metres installed in some areas for the electronic reading of electricity and gas are causing health problems for householders. These apparently are becoming compulsory in a lot of areas.

Today we have multiple TVs, mobiles and a host of other electronic equipment in our homes. TVs get bigger and bigger and there are more and more gadgets coming on the market.

There is a lot of information and evidence regarding emissions from the above appliances and others, such as children's electronic games and other household equipment. The emissions and radiation from these are no doubt harmful to health. I hope this awareness encourages you to take precautions to protect yourself and your family as much as possible in this ever increasing world of technology.

SUMMARY OF STEP 5

- Use natural chemical free products for all cleaning and laundry, including clothes, towels and bed linen

- Eliminate mould from your home, whether it be from dampness in a room or under the home, or in pillows, mattresses, carpets etc.

- Do not use aluminium or plastic for cooking or storage of food

- Minimise EMFs in your home, i.e. all electrical appliances including kitchen, games, TVs, microwave ovens, telephones, computers and mobiles.

CHAPTER 7

STEP 6
FIRST AID – HELP YOURSELF WITH KITCHEN CUPBOARD AND NATURAL REMEDIES

Disclaimer – These remedies are not in place of medical advice. It is recommended that if you are not sure about symptoms or a problem is persistent, do not hesitate to get medical advice.

The purpose of this section is merely to highlight that there are many remedies for first-aid use. If we help ourselves a little more and not run for a prescription for every sniffle and ache we will help prevent overuse of medications, help save our doctors precious time for more urgent consults and protect our immune system at the same time.

My search for nature's remedies (not out of a factory) started when my children were born to protect them and their immune systems from unnecessary medications. I use the same basic 'natural' first-aid kit today which I started almost 30 years ago. I just add to it as I go along and learn more. I thought I knew everything when I was in my twenties but now as a grandma I embrace each day as another opportunity to learn something else and there is so much to know.

I emphasise this is for first-aid purposes and NOT to be used in place of medical checks and advise when you feel it necessary. Only at onset of symptoms or when you are certain of what you are dealing with should these suggestions be tried. If anything is persistent or getting worse, consult a doctor.

As I mentioned previously my favourite 'emergency' kit is homeopathic which we also carry with us when travelling and which we have used for a long time and has always proven extremely helpful to us. Most of these can be purchased in health stores or even online.

HOMEOPATHIC REMEDIES

REMEDY	SYMPTOMS PHYSICAL
ARSENICUM ALB	Sickness, diarrhoea, stomach ache
ALIUM CEPA	Common cold, sneezing, runny nose etc
ACONITE	anything sudden – sore throat, cold, headache
ARNICA also cream apply externally but not on open wounds	After injury, bruising, air sickness, before and after surgery, dentist, stops haemorrhage, prevents DVT when travelling, boils, bedsores insomnia due to overtiredness
BELLADONNA	anything red hot, swollen, throbbing earache, throat, headache, mumps, abscess, sunburn
APIS MEL	stings, itching-swelling, allergic reactions cystitis
GELSENIUM	flu like symptoms, jet lag, weary aching muscles
BRYONIA	anything dry - throat, cracked lips, sore breasts
NUX VOMICA	nervous indigestion or effects of overeating or over drinking, vertigo, travel sickness, cystitis
MERC SOL	toothache, earache, abscesses
CARBO VEG	flatulence, loss of voice, nausea, vertigo cold feet

HYPERICUM	repairs nerve endings, especially coccyx, wounds after operations, spasms after injury, tingling burning, numbness
RHUX TOX	prickly heat, herpes, sciatica, rheumatism
EUPHRASIA	Hay fever, streaming eyes, runny nose, light sensitivity, worse indoors in warmth

KITCHEN CUPBOARD REMEDIES FOR EVERYDAY AILMENTS

THROAT, EAR AND CHEST INFECTIONS

Some remedies to try.

- Cut onion in half and leave by the bedside overnight
- Boil an onion in milk and drink before sleeping – gets rid of mucus in the system
- Cut up onion and cover in honey – the juices will combine to make a cough syrup which can be taken anytime – breaks up the most stubborn coughs and helps bring up mucus
- Take the pip out of the onion and place in the outer ear canal – you can also use garlic – calms down inflammation and sooths pain
- Chop a white onion in half, cup half the onion in the hand and cup over the nose and inhale 2-3 times and breathe out through the mouth into the open air
- For colds and flu put a couple of heaped tablespoonfuls of mustard powder in a bowl of hot water and soak your feet for 10-15 minutes before you go to bed. This will sweat the cold out of you. Repeat every evening as necessary

SORE THROATS

- Gargle with either sea salt or Himalayan rock salt in water, several times throughout the day to kill infection. In between take a tsp of raw honey also to kill infection but also to sooth the lining of the throat
- A level tsp of glycerine at bedtime stops the throat from tickle during the night

- Put one tsp dried sage in a mug and pour over boiling water. Allow to cool, strain and gargle with liquid several times throughout the day
- Fresh ginger – a natural antiseptic. This can be chewed to clean the mouth, for gum infections etc., or can be sliced and added to water to drink

CONSTIPATION

- The problem is probably the diet – make changes, eat more fibre and fresh fruit and vegetables
- Take one tsp sesame seeds with sip of water 20 minutes before food and drink every morning
- A slice of lemon in hot water on going to bed and first thing upon rising
- Massage lower abdomen around naval and below in a clockwise movement for constipation; anti-clockwise for diarrhoea

HEADACHES

- If the pain is in the eyes, forehead and front head this can be attributed to the digestive system. Check what you have eaten, say last two meals, and keep a diary note for reoccurring headaches and see if the same food is the problem
- Headache at the back of the head is often related to the spine, or tension.
- Migraines can be related to spine/neck. Have a chiropractor check your alignment. Try eating eight raw almonds including the skin to relieve migraines and also try one of the homeopathic remedies mentioned earlier
- *DIGESTIVE – put half tsp aluminium free bi-carbonate soda in cup, pour on a little boiling water from kettle, it will fizz, cool with a little cold water and drink. This sometimes can help your headache by clearing your system. You can do this two or three times a day but only as a quick remedy not to be repeated often or it can do more harm than good
- FOOD POISONING – homeopathic remedy – arsenicum alb for any of the following symptoms; headaches, nausea, vomiting, stomach pain (follow instructions on label). Activated charcoal is also excellent to help clean out the system from infection

INDIGESTION some suggestions

- *Bi-carbonate of soda as per instructions above for upset stomach with food or over-eating
- The cause can be fermentation of food from poor elimination
- Or take one tsp of caraway seeds with a little water to remove gas.
- Sipping warm water and putting a water bottle on the abdomen may help – cold drinks may cause contraction which can exasperate the problem
- The homeopathic remedy carbo veg is good for gas and acidity.

DIARRHOEA

- Grated raw apple for children to eat as pectin helps coagulate the stool
- Arrowroot or even cornflour can help as a drink or mixed into food
- Cottage cheese helps bind loose bowels
- If caused by food poisoning see remedies above

BABIES

For gripe pains, teething pain, calming and settling a baby.

Chamomile. Either the homeopathic remedy – follow instructions or advice of homeopath – or you can also dip a chamomile teabag in some boiled cooled water to make a drink. Mothers drinking chamomile tea will pass on the help via the breast milk

GENERAL FATIGUE

Likely cause is the body low on minerals. Take one tsp molasses three times a day. This is full of natural iron, calcium, potassium, phosphorus, sulphur, some zinc and minor minerals as well. The body assimilates this well because it is natural. Diet should always be considered in severe instances

Drink nettle tea three times a day. Nettle is full of iron and minerals!

Often with such fatigue the body has been depleted of enough vital nutrients over a long period of time caused by being too busy to eat, skipping meals, snacking, using up endless energy without replacing it. Just starting to eat better isn't going to resolve this overnight. The body needs to catch up, get in front with energy and nutrients so when the person exerts, it is not exhausting the total supply every time. Therefore nutritional saturation is necessary and as much rest and relaxation as possible to allow the body to recover. I have a couple of clients with this problem. They can feel great when they are eating regularly and taking time out but as soon as they commence their crazy non-stop lifestyle they are exhausted and again they are not giving their body time to get in front. How difficult it is to eat nutritious food/drink six times a day when dashing here and there all day! You have to find a way – and you can!

HOME-MADE COUGH AND COLD SYRUPS

Onion & Honey

Peel and chop an onion, put in a dish and cover with raw honey and leave covered for a few hours. The onion juice and honey will merge into watery syrup. Drain off and put into a clean covered jar and keep in the fridge for up to a week. Onion and honey are very potent anti-viral and anti-bacterial and will help clear throat and respiratory system of symptoms. Take one teaspoonful three times a day or as often as is needed.

Raspberries, salt and glycerine

Put a bag of fresh, frozen preservative-free frozen raspberries into a sieve, over a dish. When the raspberries thaw the juice will flow into the dish –it helps to stir and mash a little. Extract as much juice as possible and put into a clean jam jar in the fridge. A little raw sugar can be added as a preservative and sweetener. When making the cough syrup add one level teaspoon of glycerine, a few grains of a natural salt and about three tbsps raspberry syrup and mix altogether. Take one tsp three times a day or as often as is needed.

Children love these toxic-free remedies.

BLOCKED SINUSES

Gently rubbing glycerine down the bridge of the nose helps unblock sinuses.

Also cup the hand and put cold water in it, place one finger over one nostril and sniff the water vigorously up the other nostril. A few grains of natural fine salt can be added to the water.

HAYFEVER

Dip a cotton bud in glycerine or castor oil and circle around the inside of each nostril, the sticky oil will prevent particles and pollen entering the nose.

BI-CARBONATE OF SODA

There are whole books written about this wonderful product both for health remedies and toxic-free cleaning in the home.

Bi-carbonate of soda is alkalising, and applying the principle of Dr Otto Warburg's statement that no disease can survive in an alkalised environment, bi-carb can be a quick temporary fix for a few things. So as well as taking it orally occasionally for upset stomach and to help flush out our digestive system, or to quickly alkalise our system if we have a cold or flu, we can use it for many other things too numerous to mention here.

Examples

Mouthwash – mix with a little water and gargle.

Cleaning teeth. Make into a paste (you can add other ingredients to make your own toothpaste).

Dab on cold sores and mouth ulcers

Sprinkle in shoes as a deodoriser, especially in summer.

Pat under arms to deodorise

CASTOR OIL AND ITS MANY USES

These are too numerous to mention but here are some examples. The castor oil must be organic best quality, cold pressed for maximum healing potential.

I reiterate again, natural remedies are not cures; often other issues have to be addressed, mainly diet.

Constipation. Take one tsp of castor oil a day in milk or juice as a gentle purgative. In addition, castor oil can be massaged into the lower abdomen depending on severity of the problem (don't forget the sesame seed remedy too).

Earache: Sometimes a couple of drops in the ear can often arrest infection.

Skin: Acne, sun spots, eczema etc. Try one tsp a day for a few days to help clean the colon and also apply the oil to the skin.

Arthritis: Massage oil into calcifications morning and night consistently for as long as it takes and it can break down the calcification.

Hair: Massage into the scalp to encourage hair growth.

Immune system enhancement: Castor oil compresses put on the liver and abdomen have shown to boost the immune system as well as support better digestion, enhance liver function etc.

(Recommended reading "The Oil that Heals" by William A McGarey M.D)

INSTRUCTIONS FOR CASTOR OIL PACKS

Castor oil packs can be used on swollen or stiff joints and can help promote healing.

To Make the Pack

Take a piece of wool flannel and fold it into three thicknesses. Put it in a dish and pour castor oil on it. Saturate the whole flannel and leave it until it is well-saturated. When you use it, you want it saturated, but not dripping. After each use, you will probably need to add a little more castor oil. You can use the pack many times. When you're not using it, you can store it in a plastic bag in the refrigerator – it will keep for about a week.

Using the Pack

Place the pack over the area required. Then put cling film over the whole soaked pad to help avoid dripping, and then put an old towel over that. Use the pack in the evening, as you are resting before bed. Then place a heat pack over the top and keep the temperature up, so have two on the go if necessary. A wheat bag type will do, and if you don't have anything try a couple of plastic water bottles with hot tap water as heat pads. Obviously you can't put boiling water in or it would melt the bottle.

Keep the pack on for 1-1½ hours.

Make up a solution of baking soda in warm water and use paper towels or a sponge with the baking soda solution to clean off the castor oil. You might also want to take a shower with soap after that.

Use the pack for three days in a row. Then take a break for four days and repeat.

I always emphasise to clients that 'natural healing' is slow but sure, so perseverance is the key.

LAVENDER – BURNS

We cannot end this section without mentioning the healing properties of aromatic oils. This is a huge subject in itself. Whilst healing with oils goes back to ancient times, the modern day 'discovery' of their properties was instigated by a French cosmetic chemist. The story goes that a chemist working in his laboratory burnt his arm very badly and thrust it into the nearest liquid. It dramatically reduced the pain and did not blister or scar – that liquid was lavender. He spent the rest of his life researching the remarkable healing properties of nature's oils and it was from this that the modern day 'aromatherapy' was born.

One which sits in our kitchen and bathroom cupboard all of the time is lavender. Lavender is probably the most versatile of these oils. A couple of drops of lavender on your pillow or in your bath water can help promote a good night's sleep. For headaches it is helpful to put a small amount on your middle finger tips and dap on your temples and eyebrows at the bridge of the nose. To apply it to the skin after those little burns we women sometimes can get whilst cooking is a must. We know aloe Vera is also very good in this instance but I put lavender at the top of my list. A friend had such a burn and she didn't mention it to me for several hours afterwards, it may even have been the next day, and it was still painful. I introduced her to the lavender treatment and she was so impressed how quickly it took the pain away and healed she passed the information on to many other friends.

CHAPTER 8

MORE CASE STUDIES

I must reiterate again, medical advice should always be sought if you don't know what you are dealing with and if a problem persists.

TUMMY BUGS

I remember once when a really bad tummy bug was going around at school, children and teachers who caught it would be off school for about a week recovering. Yes my children did get it, and at the same time. At the first on-set of symptoms I gave them the homeopathic remedy arsenicum album 6c following the 'emergency remedy' instructions then continuing with three times a day. They very soon stopped the vomiting and diarrhoea and by the end of the first full day wanted to eat again. They returned to school a day and a half later. Their teachers asked how my children could recover so quickly when other pupils and staff were off school for a week. Of course I eagerly shared the remedy with the teacher. This is one remedy I would not travel without, over some 30 years of using it, it has never failed to help us.

Some years later after my daughter finished university she came to Australia travelling for a year (which lasted 18 months and resulted in the whole family moving here)! A few months into her trip I had a telephone call from a relative of a friend she was travelling with saying our daughter was very sick with a tummy bug. I immediately rang her in Melbourne where she was staying with a family for a while. She said someone had gone out to get a doctor as she had continuous vomiting and diarrhoea for two days and was becoming dehydrated. I reminded her that I had given her a homeopathic travel kit which she had forgotten about, and asked her to take the arsenicum alb every 15 minutes for two hours when I would call back. Two hours later the vomiting had stopped and she was well on the way to recovery. A few days later the lady of the house asked to speak with me. She explained that our daughter had caught this bug from babysitting for someone and that it had spread through the family – she had been very concerned about our daughter and the severity of the symptoms and was amazed at the speed of recovery after taking the remedy. Apparently, as the rest of the family started with the symptoms she gave them all the arsenicum at the onset which 'nipped it in the bud' and they all avoided the serious symptoms experienced by the rest. She asked me what this miracle remedy was.

A few years ago I was holidaying with family when I received an urgent call from someone who used to work for me. Please can you help us she asked, my husband has been sick for days with a tummy bug and nothing seems to help and now I have it too. I suggested they both do the following:

Boil the water in a kettle, put a level teaspoon of bi-carbonate of soda in a cup, pour on boiling water until the mixture fizzes, cool with cold water to approximately half a cup and drink it. I suggested they do these two or three times during the day. Meanwhile, I suggested she get the remedy arsenicum alb from the health store and take as directed for emergency treatment, and then continue three times a day until symptoms subside.

I received a text the next day saying all okay, both recovering well.

GOUT

I worked with a gentleman who was a gout sufferer – but he was happy to take his anti-inflammatories when he had an attack. He was not receptive to my 'natural' suggestions. One day however, after six weeks of pain and swelling and unable to get his shoes on and getting no relief from his anti-inflammatories, he surrendered and asked what he needed to do.

Well, of course dietary changes are necessary to eliminate this condition, removing stimulants like alcohol, tea, coffee, red meats from the diet and ensuring a more alkaline environment by eating of lots of vegetables, greens etc., but as an 'emergency' situation to remove pain and swelling this is what I advised him to do.

To take one tablespoon of potato juice three times a day until the swelling subsides then reduce gradually to one tablespoon a day then stop. This is achieved by peeling a potato (preferably organic), grating it into a dish with the smallest side of a grater. This will create a lot of juice if it is a good quality potato. The mixture is then pressed through a tea strainer into a cup to separate the juice from the grated potato. This can be covered and kept in the fridge for the day's dosage. Dosage must not be exceeded. The mulched potato can be used as a compress on the swelling too.

By the fourth day the swelling had reduced and the gentleman could get his shoes back on. On the fifth day the feet were back to normal. As I said, long-term changes to the diet are required to eliminate this condition altogether.

Potato is anti-inflammatory and potato poultices can be used for example on swollen joints in respect of arthritis, on the throat in respect of a sore swollen throat.

ARTHRITIS AND JOINT PROBLEMS

Changes in diet are imperative for such conditions of the body. Therefore, the advice in the early chapters of this book are a must, as well as extra help from 'natural remedies'.

Many decades ago I was introduced to MSM (methylsulfonylmethane) – an organic form of sulphur. I read the book called *The Miracle of MSM* and was amazed at the results of using this natural food supplement. Along with dietary changes it was renowned for 'getting people with arthritis out of wheelchairs'.

Firstly, let me tell you a little about this amazing food supplement.

'We need bio-available organic sulphur to live. With our current western "highly processed" diet, we typically don't get nearly enough. Sulphur is the third most abundant mineral in the body. Most abundant is calcium, then phosphorus. Sulphur is highly water soluble, and hence easily lost in sweat, urination and defecation. The body needs a constant flow of sulphur coming in, in order to function properly. Without sufficient sulphur in our bodies, we eventually suffer from an array of crippling diseases.'
Early work by Dr Stanley Jacobs indicated that DMSO, another form of sulphur, could aid the body in fighting disease. His experiments included tests with animals using DMSO on cancer, arthritis and a variety of other

inflammatory and auto-immune diseases. He had startling success. You can read about his experiments and findings in his book (also available on this website) called The Miracle of MSM.

Information: MSM Australia and MSM - Medical Information Foundation

Sulphur deficiencies can be associated with slow wound healing and many health problems. The body is in a constant state of self-repair, but we need to provide it with all the nutrients it needs to repair efficiently.

Apart from having using this supplement for myself and my family occasionally for a 'top up' and health prevention, I have recommended it to lots of people with joint problems (in its pure form). You may notice in health stores capsules for joint problems are sold with glucosamine and MSM in some proportion but such small amounts are not as effective.

The following is an example of how 'natural' treatments can help arthritis and joint problems:

ARTHRITIS

Case study one

I had a request for information for arthritis from a gentleman on behalf of his wife who apparently was in constant pain with arthritis in her neck, spine and limbs. He told me she could no longer garden, walk the dog or do any activities.

Having been satisfied that this lady was on a good diet, I recommended she take MSM supplement building up to two teaspoonsful a day in water or juice (you can take quite a lot more than this dose apparently). In addition, I introduced them to organic castor oil treatment as mentioned in the remedies section.

In ancient times castor oil was named Palma Christie (the Palm of Christ), because of its amazing healing properties. I mentioned at the beginning of the book how I used it on my hand after the doctor had recommended surgery!

I recommended she massage the castor oil into the painful areas of her body and, in addition, on three consecutive days a week to do a compress treatment.

Several weeks later I spoke with the husband who said we are not telling anybody because it is too good to be true but my wife woke up this morning and had no pain for the first time in two years. The lady in question is back doing all the things she used to do. Sometime later her husband told me that a large calcification she had on her knee for ten years had disappeared.

Dietary changes are of course extremely important. Treatments such as these can help tremendously but if we are looking at prevention then other changes have to be made. There are also other things which can help the pain of arthritic joints like arnica creams and gels, MSM, potato poultices and many others.

Case study two – back injury

A friend hurt her back in recent months. She was in a lot of pain and taking painkillers all day. A week or so later there was no improvement, even though she was having physiotherapy. I strongly advised that she should have an x ray, but preferably through a chiropractor, which she did. After her consultation for the results of the x ray she called me. I could tell in her voice that it was not good news. I have never before heard a chiropractor say that he couldn't help and that someone would probably need surgery! The diagnosis was severe spinal degeneration and there were also bone spurs present. Being a very active lady indeed she was devastated and depressed and was envisioning life in a wheelchair. I assured her that there were some things we could try before resorting to surgery. Following an oil compress of St John's Wort oil on three consecutive days, (this treatment can help 'cushion' injuries and take the pressure away), I suggested she massage her lower back (where the pain was) with organic castor oil every morning and night consistently. This would help break up the bone spurs and promote healing. The next most important thing was to take MSM sulphur to help the body 'rebuild and repair'. As my friend was on a very good diet, we didn't have to focus on food on this occasion.

I explained that consistency and perseverance were necessary for results. You cannot expect long standing deterioration to repair overnight. It took around three weeks for the pain to completely go, and for her to be able to walk comfortably. She has continued this treatment now for several months. She recently moved house, she has been bending, packing, lifting, and climbing stairs with no back problems whatsoever. She told me she was amazed, but knew it was the continuing treatment that was responsible.

ILL HEALTH & AMALGAMS

A few years ago I met a lady who had lung cancer. She was only in her forties and had never smoked. The tumour had doubled in size in the three months since diagnosis, in spite of her efforts with change of diet. She had been advised to have her lung removed. We set about eliminating toxic foods/additives from her diet and naturally increasing more nutritious foods. Six weeks later at her next scan the tumour had stopped growing and her 'doctor' advised her to keep doing whatever it was she was doing. The next thing I strongly recommended was removal of her amalgams. It has become very common knowledge in recent years how toxic mercury is to the whole body. She followed the advice and the detoxing regime recommended by the dentist. At her next scan the tumour had started to shrink. This is another example how the toxins from all avenues of life today affect our health so adversely.

MONOSODIUM GLUTAMATE

A gentleman had constant migraines and relied on painkillers and also had a problem with a stiff knee which had been an issue for a couple of years. I suspected the culprit was food additives and in particular MSG. On the fourth day of removing foods containing these from his diet he had no problems with his knee (which he had assumed was arthritis), and also realised he was no longer having headaches.

Again, the potential side effects of this flavour enhancer are common knowledge.

Early one morning a young member of staff came into my office very upset and worried about her mother. She said her mum had another debilitating headache. It was 8.30 in the morning and she was wearing sunglasses. She asked if I could help. I called the mum and asked the mum what she had eaten the previous night and also the lunchtime of the previous day. Both meals contained several meat products which I know contained MSG. I gave her advice on how to flush her system. She avoided MSG from then on and her very bad headaches stopped.

Another young family member was having headaches and joint problems – after checking his diet, much of which was pies, sandwiches and food he ate when he was out and about working. All of these foods would contain MSG and other additives. Once avoided, his symptoms did not persist.

IgA AUTO IMMUNE DISEASE

This disease, in its final stage, results in kidney failure which requires a kidney transplant or dialysis.

I had worked with a young woman interstate who was in the initial stages of this disease and it was very quickly arrested with diet. Some years later I was approached by a gentleman who had had the disease for some 14 years, and declining. He also had osteoporosis, gout and high blood pressure. (Coincidence or not the three types of drugs he was taking for the latter three problems all listed a rare but serious side effect as kidney failure!!)

Within one month of a total change of diet the gentleman in question had stabilised kidneys for the first time in 14 years, his blood pressure readings were normal, he had experienced no gout attacks – and decided to gradually stop all medications. This is a quote from part of his last communication to me giving permission to use his case in my teachings and writing.

In 2001, doctors in Tahiti discovered that I have renal insufficiency (IgA) because of my mother's kidney disorder history. I was treated with medications accordingly.

In 2012 I was diagnosed also with apnea disorder. My weight was around 78kg to 84kg and I enjoyed social drinking, wine and beer.

After moving back to Australia I decided to reduce my intake of tablets which was six a day. I went to health food events and met Jasmine Makings in March 2014. I made an appointment with her.

After a food assessment, Jasmine gave me advice on how to eat properly, eating and drinking heaps of green vegetables, no meat for the first three months, every morning drinking a glass of water with lemon to flush out or reduce inflammation in my body and stop eating processed food. I followed her advice seriously.

I went back to Tahiti for holidays and at the same time I took the opportunity to have a complete check up with my usual doctors (general practitioner, cardiologist, nephrologist and others). They were all surprised of my blood test results. All levels went down or back to normal, also weight reduced, whilst looking and feeling really fit.

After the two months holiday, eating and drinking anything and everything, I then returned to Australia I had a major gout attack like never before. I was in agony.

I then went back on the greens and followed Jasmine's advice on nutrition once again.

Now I weigh 73kg (12/11/14) and only take one tablet for my blood pressure which is reduced to 5mg instead of 10mg of Ramipril. I have also started paddling on an outrigger canoe three times a week.

Looking and feel great!

WOUND HEALING

A gentleman working at our home was wearing a bandage around his lower leg. When I inquired what was the matter with his leg, he informed me that two years previous a vein had burst and the wound would not heal. The doctor had been treating him with antibiotics and other treatments over the two years but nothing worked. I asked him if he would try a 'natural remedy'. I told him, after showering after work every day, to clean the wound with witch-hazel after which he was to apply castor oil and cover for the night and if he was working the next day, to keep the dressing on. He was to repeat this treatment twice a day if possible. When he was in a clean environment I also asked him to expose his leg to the fresh air. When I bumped into the gentleman at a friend's house a couple of months later he told me his wound had healed. Witch-hazel is perhaps well known as a cleanser toner for cosmetic purposes, it is also an ingredient in eyewashes, but perhaps it is not realised that it can be used to cleanse wounds, including those on animals. Castor oil of course seals and heals the wound.

IRRITABLE BOWEL SYNDROME

I was asked by a lady if I could help as her symptoms had got much worse in spite of her good diet. Following a dietary assessment (and she was on a very good diet), the only thing which stood out to me was that she was eating a lot of nuts in various forms and dishes and also a lot of coconut oil. If felt she was having an excess of each and asked her to eliminate both from her diet for at least one week preferably two, then reintroduce them gradually but not in such large amounts. This is a good example of 'having too much of a good thing'. This was from her response to me.

> *My gut issues (IBS type symptoms) had slowly been getting worse again over the last few months and I was fearing the worst.*
>
> *Jasmine reviewed my diet and suggested I do a two-week elimination of nuts and coconut both of which had become a major part of my diet without me really noticing that I was eating significant amounts of these foods each day.*
>
> *During the elimination my symptoms went to the other extreme, but Jasmine suggested a few more tweaks and I have slowly started the reintroduction of nuts and coconut back into my diet.*
>
> *I really was amazed at how quickly my body reacted to the changes in diet, showing me that my symptoms really were related to what (or how much of certain foods) I was eating and my system needed a break, even though they were healthy foods you really can have too much of a good thing!*

In respect of IBS and other bowel, digestive and inflammatory disorders in this area I cannot speak highly enough of the food supplement Slippery Elm Food. This wonderful help food/remedy has been around for thousands of years. It is a powder and can be taken in water or fruit juices for a simple stomach upset or in the case of such as IBS and other inflammatory bowels diseases it can be taken daily. Slippery Elm lines acts as an internal bandage allowing tissue to heal, as a poultice drawing out heat and as a food when convalescing.

CLOSE

If you follow the guidelines given in this book, you will very soon feel the benefit. Better health for you and your family. I suggest you read the whole book through then begin again at Step 1. Make adjustments one meal at a time if you cannot manage a total change all at once. As I mentioned at the beginning of the book, the six steps followed a six-week workshop so that each one attending had a full week to implement the changes ready to move to the next step. Even when we arrived at Step 4 onwards, the participants were still working on steps one and two. It isn't all going to happen overnight unless you make very radical changes, but you can feel almost overnight benefits even with small changes initially. Remember the young mum with the eight-year-old child? In one week the symptoms had gone. The gentleman with the stiff knee, the fourth day it had gone. The other little girl mentioned earlier in the book had major changes in just over a weekend. All you have to do is make the decision to make the changes and you will never look back.

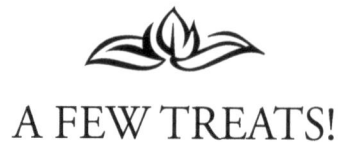

A FEW TREATS!

Welcome to my world of good health and happiness with it.

Jasmine

This small section is just to show that cutting out the bad foods doesn't mean you can't have treats. There are some fabulous recipes for the sweet tooth which are healthy and easy to make.

When I have mentioned to clients and to audiences I was writing a book, they asked if I would include recipes and I said no. I wanted to focus on re-educating – a permanent change to the way people think regarding their food and diets. They insisted I include at least some of what I shared with them. So below is a few examples of recipes I share with my clients to help them make adjustments – and an occasional treat too. There are so many healthy recipes you can access on the internet; I wish to give just a few tasters!

QUICK AND EASY CHOCOLATE NUT TREAT

RECIPE

1 cup raw pecan nuts

1 cup medjool dates (remove pips – soak for a while in water if they aren't moist).

1/4 cup cacao powder

NB If the mixture is not sticking together after processing add either a little honey or maple syrup and pulse – the mixture needs to be tacky but not wet.

METHOD

Place the pecans in a food processor and pulse until you have the texture of breadcrumbs.

Add the rest of the ingredients and pulse until combined.

Roll into balls.

Or press mixture into a square dish lined with baking paper (so it comes out easily).

Pop in fridge for ½hr then cut into slices, wrap in baking paper and put in an airtight container.

This will last many days in the fridge or freezer in an airtight container.

ALTERNATIVE RECIPE

I usually make double this recipe and also vary it e.g. –

1 cup dates

1 cup cranberries

1 cup pecans

1 cup hazelnuts or almonds

½ cup cacao powder

Add a little honey or maple as needed to bind together

HOME-MADE ICECREAM

RASPBERRY

2 cups frozen raspberries

1 raw egg white

2 tablespoons sheeps' yogurt

1 tablespoon raw honey

Blend altogether in a powerful blender. You may have to stop regularly to stir. When it is all mixed put in dish and keep in the freezer.

BANANA & MACADAMIA

3 frozen bananas

1 handful macadamia nuts

(Optional ½ tbsp of sheeps' yogurt)

Blend altogether until creamy, put in dish and keep in freezer.

NB: Sometimes you have to keep stopping and stirring these until the fruit starts to thaw a little which makes blending easier.

HUMMUS

1 can organic chickpeas rinsed and dried

Juice of 2 lemons/2 garlic cloves

2 tbsps olive oil

Pinch cayenne pepper

3 tablespoons tahini paste

Salt and black pepper

Process chickpeas in a food processor/blender to a smooth puree, add lemon juice, garlic, olive oil, cayenne and tahini and blend until creamy. Add a little extra olive oil if too thick.

NUT CREAM CHEESE

Enjoy with celery/carrots as a dip, or on crackers or toast or serve on vegetables

3 cups cashews

Juice of 2 large or 3 medium lemons

Juice of 1 lime

3-4 shallots (include some of the green stem)

½ tsp sea salt

(Filtered water as necessary)

Blend all the above ingredients to a smooth paste adding the nuts gradually. Add filtered water gradually if necessary to make blending easier, stirring regularly to achieve the desired consistency.

As my clients love my concoctions of soup – I thought I would share these as well.

SOUP RECIPES

Please note use potato or sweet potato as a thickener in all soups rather than have to add flour which is no good! I also stir in a teaspoon of molasses after cooking to add extra minerals.

BROCCOLI AND SWEET POTATO

3 large sweet potatoes peeled and chopped

1 large or 2 medium onions finely chopped

1 -2 cloves of garlic (optional)

2 large broccoli florets using all but the hard bottom root.

Sea salt, black pepper

METHOD

Cook chopped onions and garlic for a few minutes in a little butter.

Add a kettle full of boiling water.

Add chopped sweet potatoes and all broccoli.

Bring to boil and immediately simmer for about 20 minutes.

(Simmer on as low a heat as possible whilst just bubbling otherwise over heating will destroy nutrients – bear this in mind for all soups SIMMER.)

When cooked, stir in about 2 tspns of salt and a shake or two of black pepper. You can also add a level teaspoon of molasses at this stage for extra minerals.

When ready you can puree to make a thick soup. To make it creamier you can either liquidise a handful of raw organic cashew nuts with the soup or when you serve the soup add a small teaspoon of sour cream in the middle of each dish.

CAULIFLOWER SOUP

Exactly same as above. Can also use white potatoes for a change.

SPICY VEGETABLE SOUP

For this recipe you can use what vegetables you like. I generally use –

2 large onions

Pumpkin

Green beans

Garlic

Sweet potato

Cauliflower and broccoli

1 red pepper

4 ripe tomatoes (this adds flavour)

Spices (1 level tablespoon turmeric, 1 teaspoon cumin powder, ¼ tsp sweet paprika as this is hot (add a little more if you want it hotter).

Sometimes add a tin of organic lentils or chickpea for protein (or dried red lentils are quick and good without having to soak them).

You can add frozen peas, but only add at the end just until the peas are unfrozen and warm – don't boil or it will destroy the zinc in the peas.

METHOD

As before cook onions and garlic in a little butter for a couple of minutes. Add boiling water, all vegetables except peas and all spices. Bring to boil and simmer for about 20 minutes until all soft. Switch off heat and add some salt, pepper and molasses.

ENJOY!

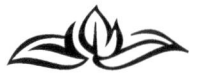

To everyone,
My best wishes
For your good health
And longevity
Jasmine x

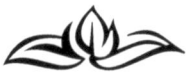

References

Dr Dwight Lundell - The Cholesterol Lie

Dr Andrew Lockie - A Family Guide to Homeopathy

Mr Jeffrey Smith GMO DANGERS

Bill Statham - The Chemical Maze,

Firman E Bear at Rutgers University Natural Gardeners Catalogue (1995)

Canarian Weekly

William A McGarey M.D - The Oil that Heals"

MSM Australia and MSM - Medical Information Foundation

Further Reading

http://www.thefoodcoach.com.au/articles/?ATID=1&ArticleID=344

http://fluoridealert.org/content/fluoride-the-hidden-poison-in-the-national-organic-standards/

http://www.livestrong.com/article/283487-nutritional-deficiencies-adhd/

http://www.safespaceprotection.com/electrostress-from-home-appliances.aspx

http://www.sweetpoison.com

http://www.jasminemakings.com

www.ingramcontent.com/pod-product-compliance
Ingram Content Group UK Ltd.
Pitfield, Milton Keynes, MK11 3LW, UK
UKHW021309180426
11947UKWH00015B/1120